Natural Remedies:

YOUR ULTIMATE WELLNESS GUIDES

Epsom Salt, Apple Cider Vinegar, Ashwagandha & Ayurveda Essential Oils

by Elena Garcia

www.facebook.com/HolisticWellnessBooks

Table of Contents

BOOK 3

BOOK 4

Book 1:

Epsom Salt

The Miraculous Mineral

Holistic Solutions & Proven Healing
Recipes for Health, Beauty & Home

by Elena Garcia

www.facebook.com/HolisticWellnessBooks

Introduction

Welcome and thank you for taking an interest in this book. You are about to start a fascinating journey learning about the wonderful world of Epsom Salt. But not only that, you will be learning really easy, practical ways of using them to boost your health and beauty plus some other very unexpected benefits in your garden.

Dig out that packet sitting in the kitchen, or maybe even the garage shelf, that you bought a while ago. It is FULL of the most amazing benefits. If you aren't using Epsom Salt every day, there is something wrong! And the thing that most people tell me when I talk about the benefits of this fascinating power packed powder is 'I never knew you could do THAT with them.'

I shared that lack of knowledge! A while ago I looked at the dusty old packet of Epsom Salt that I'd bought ages ago in a fit of enthusiasm for something I'd read about them on Facebook. I'd apparently used them for a bit and then life took over and I forgot about them. But I must admit, like many people, I was a bit unconvinced that that white powder in the unprepossessing box could actually achieve all the claims that were being made for it. That box had cost just a few bucks and I had the suspicion that something as simple as that and not backed by extensive chemical research by scientists in white coats and coming in at a high price could actually do the job. Boy! Was I wrong!

I should have known better as a lifelong practitioner and user of natural remedies but for some reason I hadn't latched on to this little wonder product. I decided to do something about that and began to do my own 'white coat' research. It didn't take long before I was using them all the time. So in this eBook you will follow in my footsteps for a while before branching off into your own discoveries of this simple homely - but wonderful - product.

I saved money by the bucketload using them as beauty products. I saved time because they worked quickly in starting to support my health

I increased my joy in my garden a hundred-fold because so many plants appreciated the Epsom Salt treatment that they came on in leaps and bounds.

So, anything that's going to save time and money – and works well has got to be worth looking at. Turn to the first Chapter and prepare to be amazed and excited.

The way to use this book depends on if you are a big picture person, or whether you like focus and detail. The big picture people should zero in on the first chapter right away. It tells you all about the salts, their history, the various categories of help they can be used for and why they are so beneficial.

After that go to the section you are most interested in and dip in there. Gradually you will read the whole book and have many new ideas about how you can use that dusty old packet in the kitchen cupboard!

The detail people need to zero in on the section that is most relevant to them. Just concentrate on that and start trying out one idea. See if it works for you then move on to the next thing. Once you have been hooked by the Epsom Salt bug you may want to learn some of their history. That can be found in the first chapter. After that you may shift your attention to one of the other uses of Epsom Salt and work your way through that. It always helps to try out the suggestions. Only when you feel the impact in, and on, yourself do you turn into a convert and make sure that Epsom Salt is always in your cupboard and you are using it every day.

Read on and enjoy...

Free Newsletter + Bonus eBook

Before we dive into the benefits and uses of Epsom salt, I would like to offer you free access to our health and wellness newsletter. This is how you will be notified about our new books at discounted prices, bonuses and giveaways.

As a special welcome gift, you will receive a free PDF eBook with healthy alkaline-paleo recipes!

Simply visit: www.holisticwellnessbooks.com/bonus

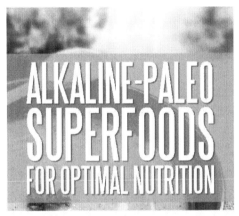

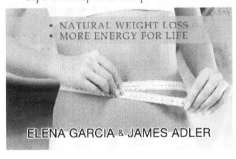

Problems with your download?

Contact us: elenajamesbooks@gmail.com

Chapter One:
The History of Epsom Salt

Once upon a time, a long time ago, there was a little village just to the south of London in England called Epsom. When I say a long time ago I mean a LONG time ago. We are going back in our time machine to the beginning of the 1600's. Four hundred years ago, to a time just after the death of Good Queen Bess (Elizabeth 1), just after the failure of Guy Fawkes in his plan to blow up the Houses of Parliament and about the time when swashbuckling Sir Walter Raleigh, explorer and colonizer of North America, bringer of tobacco to Britain and leader of the expedition to El Dorado in South America was executed. It was a turbulent time in history but through it all the little villages that spread out like plates on a tablecloth all around London went about their business and tried to stay out of the way of politics and war mongering. What they wanted was a quiet prosperous life with their families in the countryside and they went about finding ingenious ways of doing just that.

In pretty little Epsom there was a drought and a local man, Henry Wicker by name, was searching for some water for his cattle. Noticing a small trickle of water filling a hoof print in the meadows around the town he dug down a little hoping to find an underground fresh water spring. On his return after digging he discovered that indeed he had tapped into a small spring that bubbled up from the deep rocky caverns below the earth. Praising the Lord for this gift from Nature he brought his cows to the meadow and stood back to watch them drink. Imagine his surprise when they refused to take a gulp!

Exploring the water a bit more he tasted it for himself and discovered that far from being simple, pure water it was full of minerals dissolved from the rock in the caverns below and then drawn up with the power of the spring. The taste was strong and brackish so it was no wonder the cows had refused it. However Henry had been around a bit and was aware of places like Bath where the Romans had built baths for restoring their health using the hot heavily mineralized spring waters in Somerset. He began to wonder if his little trickle of 'spa' water would have the same properties and help people just as in Roman times.

He tried them out on himself and discovered that he did indeed feel better after a short while. Excitedly he began to bottle the water and sell it to the local people and dreamed of a bustling town rivaling Bath which was being refurbished in an early attempt to bring people in to sip its waters. Later, of course, Bath became very famous in the Georgian 18th Century when the beautiful elegant terraces, crescents, homes and public buildings created by Beau Nash were built to grace the town and turned it into the most desirable resort for the wealthy and high-born society people.

Little Epsom did not have such luck. The spring did not produce enough water for large public consumption although there was a short period where visitors came from as far afield as Cornwall to 'take the waters'. A triumph of good marketing on Epsom's part as the people from Cornwall actually bypassed Bath to travel all the way to the south of London Town!

By the end of the century Epsom was a busy little place with 300 beds for visitors, however the lack of a plentiful supply of the water continued to place a limit on growth. Most visitors stayed for some days, even weeks, and consumed vast quantities of the water in pint mugs. They would drink several pints in the morning then again throughout the day. In the course of a visit they could drink as much as sixteen pints!   Not surprisingly this had a significant impact on their digestion and purging, or detoxing, was the order of the day.

Despite the sinking of a second well on the other side of the town the end of Epsom Spa actually came when the pharmacists in the early 1700's discovered what was in the water that was making it so effective. From the moment that the chemical compound, $Mg_2SO_4.7H_2O$ or hydrated magnesium sulfate, was discovered poor old Epsom was doomed as the salts could now be manufactured and sold very cheaply in powder form. Soon other chemists in other parts of the country were producing the salts too and the chance to make a significant fortune was over.

However, such were Epsom Salt benefits that manufacturing of them has never stopped from that day to this and this is where we in the 21st century come in as we discover what our great, great grandparents knew.

$Mg_2SO_4.7H_2O$ **or Magnesium Sulfate**

What exactly is this?

The formula stands for a combination of hydrated magnesium, sulphur and oxygen which begins to bring us the answer as to why the compound is so effective. Right away we see that Magnesium is a significant mineral within the Salt.

Magnesium

There has been lots of research on magnesium and we know that it is a highly beneficial element in several ways to overall health. In fact it has been called the most important element in nutrition.

Among its many attributes it plays a significant role in heart health. Without it hypertension is likely to get worse and, since heart disease is a silent killer, it makes excellent sense to have your blood pressure taken regularly and if it begins to climb outside your normal range then consider if your diet is deficient in Magnesium. Proper levels of Magnesium also help Coronary Artery Disease and sufficient levels of Magnesium in the body is part of preventing hardening of the arteries and strokes.

Sulfate

The next important element in Epsom Salt formula is Sulfate. Sulfates can only be ingested through certain foods but there are not many foods that give us all the sulphate we need. Fish, organic meat, poultry, free range eggs and grass fed beef are the foods of choice for this purpose. Of course all of these are the most expensive items on a shopping list. It makes sense to have some of these high-quality sulphur carrying proteins weekly. Eating whole grains, pulses and seasonal greens most days of the week with one or two meals of high-quality organic meats will give a good balance.

For vegetarians and vegans the easiest and most pleasant ways to make sure you have sufficient sulfates are to use Epsom Salt baths regularly. The elements very readily get absorbed through your skin and enter the bloodstream rapidly. From there they find the places where they are needed and start to promote health in a variety of ways.

So why are sulfates so important?

They are what protect us from arthritis, kickstart our digestive processes by causing cascades of enzymes to start working on our food. They also help brain tissue form and are critical in the developing embryo of a baby. For example, at a point in the baby's pre-birth development sulfates are needed to build the neurones which will become the light switches in the baby's brain as they begin to grow. The neurones start connecting with one another once the infant's brain begins interacting with the outside world from the moment they are born and this is what develops a human brain.

Through a process of chemical binding it helps us detox from all kinds of contaminants, for example: drugs, heavy metals, pollution in the environment, and contamination of foods we eat. This is a vital aid to our bodies as an overloaded body full of toxins becomes sluggish and inefficient in many of the processes needed to keep you healthy. A regular detox is a good idea and suggestions for how best to do that are covered in the Health section of this book.

Why do we need Epsom Salt now more than ever?

This brings us to a relevant fact about modern diets. This is not a problem our man, Henry in Epsom would have encountered, as he did not eat a Standard Western diet with many highly processed foods. Think refined flour, sugar, margarine and dairy which tend to be part of our everyday intake. All of these work against the absorption and processing of magnesium and sulfates and leave us in a depleted state. We also tend not to eat sufficient green vegetables, plenty of nuts and oily seeds like flax to make up for what we are not able to access. This means that it can be helpful to take Magnesium supplements to boost our body levels of this vital element and to begin taking regular (3 times/week) Epsom Salt baths so that both magnesium and sulfate can be soaked into the body. The next section will show you how.

Chapter 2:
Epsom Salt Baths and Your Health

With the history of 'taking the waters' which was an annual practice for many of the gentry in Regency England the idea of creating your own 'spa' in your home has become standard for us today. However there is a long history of the practice of bathing as a health promoter. Not only England had Spa Towns, but on the Continent, where places like Baden-Baden in Germany's Black Forest welcomed European royalty to its glorious spa buildings, the idea of self-care through using natural remedies influenced a very strong tradition of alternative health in Europe too.

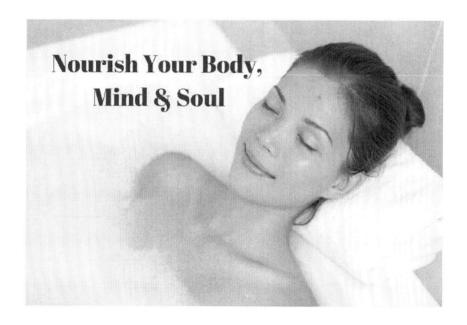

Nourish Your Body, Mind & Soul

So now it is time to go to your bathroom and look at it with fresh eyes. Think about what the spas of yesteryear had that made them so good at supporting good health and curing some ills that were not responsive to other forms of medicine.

For this we need to go back in our time machine even further into the past and visit the baths in Roman and Greek times when these civilizations were at their height.

The History of Spas and Health Care

Bathing was an incredibly important activity in Roman times and most towns had hundreds of bathing houses. The wealthy had private baths and that is the trend we have carried on in our modern homes. However the rich Romans would have had several bathing rooms, each with a different type of cleansing experience such as steaming, cold water baths or warm water baths. Do you see already how you might use your bathroom creatively to make different experiences for yourself?

Even earlier in history the Greeks started the practice of having small bathing containers for foot care and hand care. Gradually the 'containers' became larger and began holding a whole body, similar to the baths we know. The Romans however carried this even further and built baths which became large enough for many bathers to share. The whole trip to the local baths became a social event as well as a practical one for washing off the dust and keeping one's body clean. Business deals, liaisons and friendships were conducted in these public Baths and the very small cost of using the services put the baths within reach of everyone.

From entering the baths the person started with the cold water tank and progressed through tepid baths to the hottest water, then returned via a tepid bath again and there began the process of massage with oils, scraping of the skin to clean and rejuvenate it. During this they paid close attention to the condition of their bodies as they took their time to relax and regain not only a clean state of body – but also a settling and calming of their minds. In some of the best public baths they then moved on to a dry room where they could rest and relax some more before being ready to re-enter their lives.

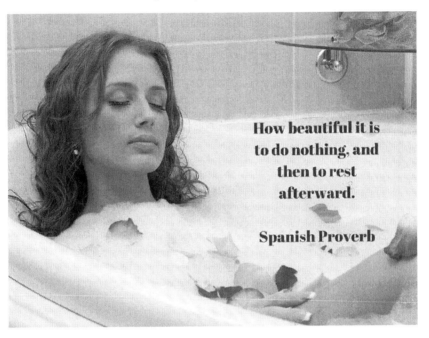

How beautiful it is to do nothing, and then to rest afterward.

Spanish Proverb

To try at home. Give yourself the time you need to make bathing and soaking an integral and necessary part of your health routine. Make it as important to you as brushing your teeth and combing your hair. Perhaps in today's world we can't do this every day, unlike the Romans, but we could have an evening a week, or a weekend morning or afternoon to devote to ourselves. Take the time to soak and adjust the temperature of the water as you lie there. Use Epsom Salt and a variety of essential oils to soak in through your skin as you lie and drift. Do not use soap as this makes the salts less effective. As the water drains use moisturizers and salves to dress any areas where you have bruises or very dry skin, then wrap yourself in a warmed fluffy towel or dressing gown and lie quietly on the bed as you dry off. This gives the salts, oils and salves the best chance to sink deeply into your tissues, easing aches and pains and healing your system.

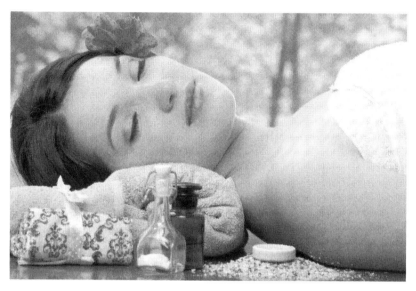

This is one of the most de-stressing ways to spend an hour (or more). If you make it a routine and insist that you have your 'me time' families grow to respect your privacy and in the end may well start to copy you!

The Romans were exceptionally civilized people and they decorated their bathing rooms in beautiful ceramics, and designs which brought the sea to mind, such as sculptures of dolphins and sea creatures. They also had the bathing areas open to the gardens and this allowed bathers to soak their senses in greenery, flowers, birdsong and gentle breezes as well as soaking up the water and minerals. All in all the Romans understood the importance of making a gorgeous sensuous experience of their ablutions and this influenced them positively at body, mind and spirit levels.

To try at home: bring plants into your bathroom. Take the trouble to bring a beautiful flower blossom into the bathroom and put it where you can quietly rest your gaze on it, noticing it's symmetry, its energy, color, scent ... This is a way to be mindful and bring in a simple meditative practice to help relieve your stress and allow your nervous system to move into 'relaxation mode' rather than the typical 'action' mode.

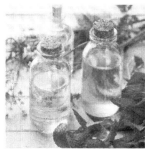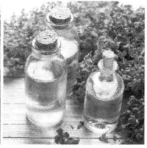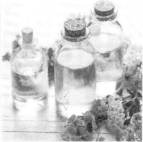

When you are buying Epsom Salt to begin your everyday use of its amazing properties be aware that there are 3 types of Epsom Salt

Don't worry, it is unlikely that you will buy the wrong type as they tend to be sold in very different stores or departments depending on the purpose you have for it.

1. Food grade or USP Grade (United States Pharmaceutical Grade) which is quality controlled and therefore pure. These are the Epsom Salt that you will find in the personal care range of products and in the grocery store. Here it will be sold in small quantities of plus/minus 500g and is likely to cost less than a bottle of shampoo.

2. Technical Grade which is for Agricultural use and is therefore a less tested and quality controlled product. Also known as Industrial Grade and can be used in mass

amounts for fertilizing. In fact it will be sold in large bags for this purpose.

3. Asian Epsom Salt which is made abroad in China or Asia and is not regulated to the same extent as those made in America or Europe. This certainly makes them cheaper but they may well have impurities in them such as heavy metals and are best avoided.

Chapter 3:
Health Tips for Epsom Salts

If you think about the body and all the extraordinary processes that are involved in being alive and being healthy we can see just what an awe-inspiring thing the body really is. We can also start to understand just how many things can go wrong if its systems get out of balance. This is why it is so important to have regular health care habits so that we service our bodies in the same way we service our cars. Preventive action is always easier and more efficient than a knee-jerk response to something going wrong.

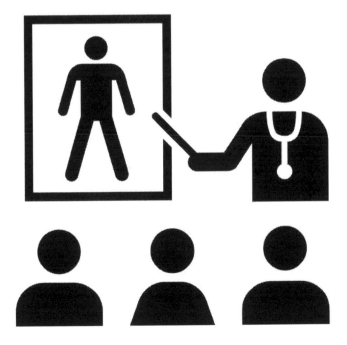

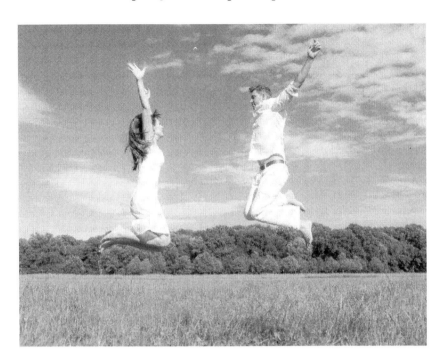

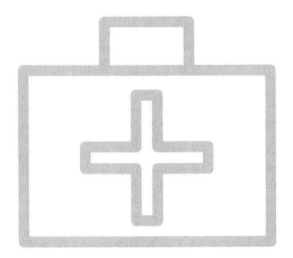

There are 10 systems in the body:

1. Cardiovascular
2. Nervous
3. Endocrine
4. Skin
5. Digestive
6. Reproductive
7. Skeletal
8. Muscular
9. Respiratory
10. Urinary

Of course, all these systems work together and support one another to make the whole body, mind and spirit healthy. However, what more than half of them have in common is that magnesium is an essential element in their efficient working. Thus directly, or indirectly, magnesium influences everything!

Sulfates too are indispensable as they work at a different level influencing the functioning of enzymes, particularly those in the stomach and digestive system, the production of amino acids which are building blocks for protein in our bodies (muscle) and forming antioxidants which help to reduce inflammation and infection.

Understanding the Body's Need for Epsom Salt and other minerals

Nervous system

Benefits: Stress reduction, sleep improvement, relief from migraine and tension headaches.

This is where magnesium eases stress and promotes deep relaxation. Low levels of magnesium lead to the body producing less serotonin. As one of the neurotransmitters responsible for our 'feel good' states we can end up low and depressed without enough of this biochemical.   If you are taking enough through the regular use of Epsom Salt your appetite will be stable, your sleep will be regular and many people report a dropping off in the frequency of migraine headaches.

Muscular system

Benefits: Relieves aches and muscle cramps.

Typical aches and pains for many people are caused by arthritis and osteoporosis which has been associated with calcium deficiency. However, without magnesium calcium cannot be absorbed properly and that can lead to one of the two types of arthritis (osteo or rheumatoid). It doesn't help to take calcium tablets alone as calcium can then collect in the tissues but still not be absorbed properly into the bloodstream and bones. Make sure that if you are taking a supplement it contains both elements. Even taking magnesium tablets alone will improve calcium take up in the body – and that might be all you need.

Cardiovascular system

Benefits: Heart protection and circulation improvement

Eases the heart and helps to prevent hardening of the arteries and stops blood clots forming. The magnesium in Epsom Salt is a powerful heart protector.   Given how prevalent heart disease is with its high blood pressure, raised cholesterol levels and disturbed eating patterns, symptoms which all point to the start of Syndrome X (metabolic syndrome) it makes sense to take preventive action early on. Have a look at your family history and if there are signs of heart disease running in the family – hypertension, heart attacks or strokes – get into the habit of taking those baths and adding in Epsom Salt to your routine right now. As a side benefit the Salt helps to improve your circulation so that if you add in some regular exercise to your routine too you are giving yourself an even better chance of protection.

Digestive System

Constipation relief, optimum use of nutrients in food

Relieves constipation and works with the digestive system to make it more efficient at absorbing nutrients from food. Because the Epsom Salt with its dosage of hydrated magnesium and sulfate helps fluid to be absorbed into the digestive tract, food waste becomes moist and it is able to pass more easily, and painlessly, along the elimination organs. It also helps to tone the cells and smooth muscle of the digestive system which mends leaky gut syndrome and helps food matter pass quickly through the different stages of digestion allowing the body to absorb the nutrients its needs rapidly.

However the ways in which Epsom Salt can help the digestive system don't stop there. The other great benefit of the Salt is that it can reduce inflammation. More people are understanding now just how inflamed our bodies can become. Mostly this is to do with our diets which stack up refined produce and keep us eating foods which bring the body tissues into a state of acidity. The acidity works on joints, muscle and at cellular levels throughout the body reducing their efficiency and seriously jeopardizing health long term. We need to make the body more alkaline to balance all that acidity and reduce the inflammation. We can do this by having a diet far heavier in leafy greens and stopping taking sugar, refined white flour and processed meats as part of our daily consumption.

The benefits of a better-balanced Ph in your body are many:

* you will recuperate more quickly from any disease,

* cuts will heal quickly and cleanly,

* bruises will fade rapidly

* bacterial infections and viral attacks will be less severe or not even start

* inflammation from sunburn will be reduced So don't forget to pack a box of Epsom Salt when you go on holiday. Make up a spray which you spritz on your exposed skin regularly, especially after a period in direct sunlight.)

* swollen areas will be reduced in size, since much of that swelling is caused by the body trying to lessen the amount of inflammation internally.

Endocrine System

Benefits: Reduces blood sugar

The endocrine system is where you secrete and balance hormones and where your needs for adrenalin, insulin, oestrogen, testosterone and other vital biochemicals are managed. As you can imagine this system is essential to feeling well and balanced. One of the most important jobs the magnesium within the Epsom Salt has is to make insulin more effective in the body. It helps the insulin in your body to be an effective blood sugar reducer.

Having the right amount of magnesium daily can reduce your blood sugar by more than 30%. The good news is that you can get a daily dose through soaking in an Epsom Salt bath as the magnesium is absorbed so readily through the skin., What an excellent excuse for that nightly 'dialing down for sleep' soak in the bath.

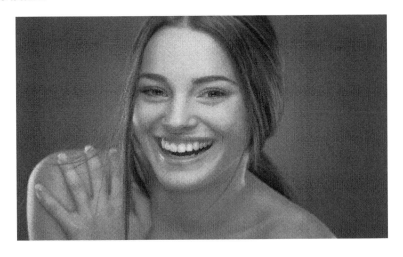

Skin, nails, hair system

Benefits: eliminate infections, cleanses, antibiotic action

A mammoth system used for protection of the whole body skin, nails and hair play a crucial part in looking after you. One of the biggest advantages of skin is that it is permeable, in other words elements such as magnesium, sulfates etc. can pass through the top layer of the skin. The elements then get absorbed into the blood and lymph systems and begin to circulate through the body finding the parts which need the minerals most. Think about how we get our daily dose of Vitamin D – straight from sunlight through our skin and into our body. This means we can use our skin to nourish ourselves at a very deep level, very easily.

You can develop some diseases of this protective layer such as a fungus which can invade the nail bed, athlete's foot which can affect the skin on the feet and toes or acne where the pores become deeply infected. All of these conditions can be treated through absorbing Epsom Salt. Use a foot bath if you are short of time or an Epsom Salt compress for your face.

Urinary System

Benefits: Detoxifies the whole body.

The urinary system is designed to carry toxins out of the body and to continually give us the equivalent of an internal wash. Some of the more dangerous things that we absorb from the food we eat, the water we drink and the air we breathe are the so-called 'heavy metals'. The ones we are most aware of are cadmium, mercury, lead and arsenic. Remember the old stories about the dandies and ladies in Elizabethan times dying from lead poisoning because they used a lead based whitening powder on their faces! Well, we don't use that now but we still have many objects in our environment that leak lead and the other metals which we end up absorbing in roundabout ways. One of the problems with heavy metals is that they tend to sink into the tissues and not be flushed out through any other system. Using Epsom Salt the heavy metals then have something else to bind with and the magnesium sulfate with its 'passenger' of heavy metal is able to be swept through the system and away. This leaves the body tissues far healthier and is an excellent way to detox.

To try at Home

Instructions for Salt Baths

All of these systems can be accessed by using Epsom salts in a bath. It is advised that this is done 3 times/week for the best benefits.

The amount of Epsom Salt to be used is at least 2 full cups of the Salt. It depends of course on how full you like your bath to be and if you are one of those people who like to float in their bath then up to 500g of Epsom Salt would work well to a tub of water.

Twelve to twenty minutes is the average amount of time to stay in the water to allow the absorption of the elements. Remember that you can also gradually increase, then decrease the temperature of the water to echo the Roman Bathing techniques. Even better is then to lie down for up to an hour while your body dries and heals as Nature intended.

If you are using a footbath as a shorter, quicker pick me up, use half a cup of Epsom Salt and let your feet soak for ten minutes before wrapping them up in a warm towel and lying down for a few more minutes.

Instructions for Epsom Salt Drinks

Bathing, although a sensuous and gorgeous way to support good health, is not the only way to obtain the benefits of Epsom Salt. Going back to our history lesson again the whole movement began with people drinking the waters. In fact in Epsom itself, at its height, visitors were drinking up to sixteen pints/day! That is quite a shock to the system. Not advised today, but the following recipes will help you with your detoxing regime and give gentle support to your liver and excretory organs.

Gentle Detox with Epsom Salt

There are some important facts to know about before you begin any detox routine. These are especially important to remember when using Epsom Salt as they are so powerful and beneficial you need to understand how to best help your body.

1. It takes two days to detox so plan to do this over a weekend or during a holiday.
2. Before you begin buy in:
   - A grapefruit (people on cardiac management medication need to check if grapefruit is safe to mix with the medicine you are taking). If you are in any doubt rather use an orange or half a teaspoon of baking soda in the mix.
   - Extra virgin olive oil.
   - Plenty of fresh filtered water to drink throughout the regime.
3. Magazines or books/videos/CD's you have been planning to get to 'sometime'.
4. Don't plan any activity during the two days – just think of them as 'Totally Me Time' and enjoy the rest.
5. The day you plan to start have a no-fat breakfast and lunch. This would be toast and honey or fruit puree, a bowl of vegetables and rice or a cereal grain like quinoa. This is done to place no extra stress on your liver.
6. Stop drinking or eating by 2 pm on your first day.

Detox Regime.

Mix together:

- 4 tablespoons Epsom Salt
- 3 cups filtered water

Instructions:
1. Store in fridge.
2. Drink your first three-quarters of a cup of Epsom Salt mix around 6 pm on Day 1. If the slightly 'soapy' taste is unpleasant for you add a squirt of lemon juice or orange juice to adjust it to suit you.

3. Drink your second three-quarters of a cup of the mixture at 8 pm. Keep resting.
4. Make up a cup of olive oil (half a cup) and grapefruit juice half a cup (or alternative) and mix together thoroughly. Let stand.
5. At 10 pm drink the oil mixture. You can flavor this if you find it hard to swallow – but gulping it down quickly to get it finished works too!
6. Rest quietly for the remainder of the night.
7. In the morning when you wake up take the next three-quarters of a cup of Epsom Salt mix.
8. Go back to bed and rest again for two hours.
9. Around 10 am take the last cup of Epsom Salt mix.
10. Rest again for 2 hours and then drink some fruit juice of your choice.
11. After half an hour you can have some lovely slices of cut up fruit such as apples, bananas, paw paw, mango.....
12. In another half hour a light meal of salad/vegetables and fish/chicken.

Dinner can be whatever you would normally have.

Do not take yourself far from the bathroom as you are likely to have a short spell of diarrhea at this point. Keep taking it easy although you can now be a bit more active since you have been eating.

Epsom Salts as a Laxative

If you don't want to go through the Detox regime but you have been suffering from some constipation, Epsom Salt helps in this case too.

Recipe:

1. Mix together 2 teaspoons of Epsom Salt in one cup of filtered water.

2. Stir it well and add some lemon juice or a teaspoon of lemon/orange or cranberry juice if you'd like to make it more palatable.
3. Drink this cupful two times/day leaving at least 4 hours between each dose.
4. As with the detox make sure you stay close to the bathroom as it can start working anytime between half an hour to six hours after drinking depending on your age, weight and type of metabolism.

Keep drinking plenty of water to keep your digestive track moist and your cells well hydrated. If it is more convenient for you - you can make up a jug of the Laxative mix by tripling the amounts above and keep it refrigerated so that you can just pour your twice daily dose from the jug at the right times. Remember to stir well each time as sometimes the Epsom Salt takes a while to dissolve.

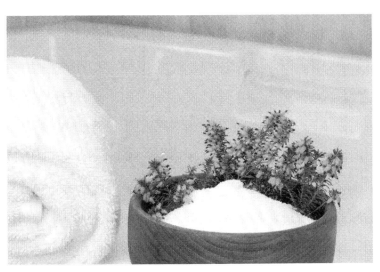

Chapter 4:
First Aid and Epsom Salt

Our Epsom Salt is such a good all-rounder that it is also an idea to keep some in a bottle in your first aid kit. The everyday cuts, bruises, stings and splinters can all be healed with the help of Epsom Salt.

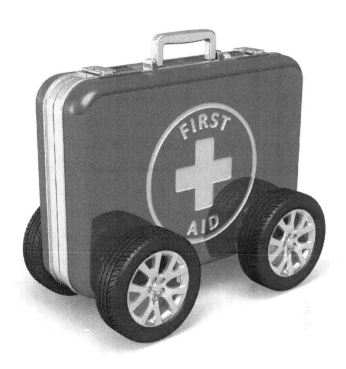

Bug bites and bee sting

Two and a half tablespoons of Epsom Salt well mixed into a cup of cold water make an excellent concentrated solution for tackling bites and stings. Pour some of the solution on a cotton pad or facecloth and keep applying to the site of the bite or sting until the redness and discomfort have died down. Remember that if you have trouble breathing after a sting you may be allergic and you need to see a doctor/hospital immediately.

Hangover

A bit of over-indulgence can leave you feeling sluggish and lethargic. These are signs of some toxicity in your body and just a quarter of a teaspoon of Epsom Salt in half a cup of warm water will settle things down. It's important to remember to drink plenty of fresh filtered water with this remedy so that you really flush your system out and keep hydrated. For better results, add some lemon or grapefruit juice. Also, avoid caffeine as it will make you even more dehydrated.

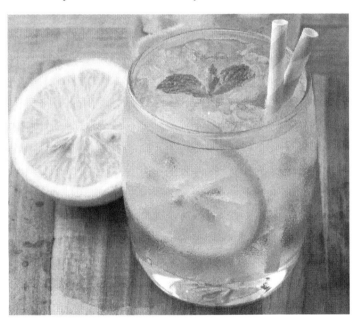

Splinter and Bruise Help

Similar to the string and bite remedy Epsom Salt can be used to reduce the swelling, inflammation and discoloration of bruises or splinters. Making a solution of two tablespoons of Epsom Salt and a cup of cold water works as an effective compress when a cloth pad is soaked in it and applied to the affected site. Keep the wet cloth on the area until it begins to warm up with the heat of your skin, then squeeze out and soak again in the solution. Apply again and keep doing this for five or six applications. This helps to combat any infection as well as the remaining inflammation.

Eye wash

Sometimes we can develop a painful stye on our eyelid or contract conjunctivitis (pink eye). Epsom Salt can come to the rescue here by making up a very mild concentration of half teaspoon Epsom Salt to a cup of blood temperature water (just tepid). Mix well so that the Salt dissolve and use as an eye bath or as a warm compress. Soak a facecloth in the weak solution and squeeze out lightly then place over the infected eye. Allow the cloth to cool slightly then keep refreshing the cloth in the solution until the discomfort in your eye lessens slightly. Keep repeating every couple of hours until you can see the improvement in the tissue.

Warts

Warts can make an unpleasant appearance on your skin and a quick and easy way to turn to natural remedies to help yourself is to mix together 1 tablespoon Epsom Salt with 4 tablespoons Apple Cider Vinegar. Keep this in the fridge and use cotton swabs to dab some onto the warts 3 – 5 times/day. Just allow the liquid to dry off itself each time which will leave a coat of solution on the warts in between treatments. Keep this up for 5 days and see how it helps them to heal.

As well as keeping a wound from a splinter free from infection Epsom Salt can also contribute to extracting the splinter itself using the power it has to draw water out of tissue. The change in osmotic pressure will help the splinter move to the surface of its own accord. Achieve this by soaking the place where the splinter is lodged in a mix of 2 tablespoons of Epsom Salt to one cup of water.

Epilepsy and MS

In the Health section we paid a lot of attention to Epsom Salt as a relaxant and as something that promotes sound sleep and stress relief. For those of you who have Multiple Sclerosis, Epilepsy, ME or asthma which can be triggered by stress it is a good idea to support yourself as much as possible by having a daily warm Epsom Health bath. The doses of Magnesium will help you sleep better and the practice of daily relaxation – especially if you enhance it through mediation or just having a quiet time in the bath – will mean that your nervous system will learn to stay in the Relaxation mode of the parasympathetic system longer each day. This will reduce the excitation of the sympathetic nervous system and make less work for your body.

Chapter 5:
Epsom Salt and Beauty

We now have a thorough understanding of the many ways in which Epsom Salt with its unique combination of magnesium and sulfate helps us to maintain our natural well-being, and correct our health issues before they get too established. Remember prevention is always better than cure. Though cure is a real bonus too!

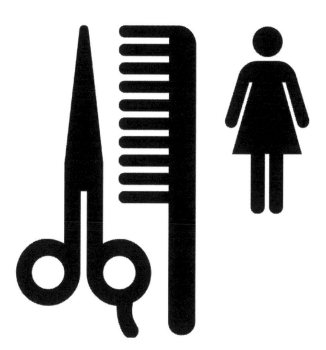

Health is bound up with Beauty and as you might expect there are many ways Epsom salts can be used to boost your beauty, and benefit your health too. In this section we will look at the best methods for using Epsom Salt as beauty aids and highlight the specific benefits each one brings.

Before we start on this section it is a good idea to check out your bathroom and kitchen cupboards for other natural products you have which can be combined with Epsom salts to make wonderful new mixtures to pamper yourself at every level.

Moisturizing cream: your favorite whatever it is:

- Essential oils – particularly peppermint, eucalyptus, lavender, thyme
- Bentonite clay
- Petroleum jelly
- Coffee grounds
- Sesame oil - extra virgin if possible
- Olive oil and coconut oil
- Tomato
- Aloe Vera gel
- Chamomile Tea (if you have fair hair)
- Black Tea (if you have dark hair)
- Favorite hair conditioner

Skin:

Exfoliation

Use Epsom salts as an exfoliating cream by adding in half a teaspoon of Salt to the usual amount of facial cleanser you use. Stir them together and apply to your face then rinse off with cool water. The cool water will act as a toner for your skin and the Epsom Salt will help to lift off the top layer of skin cells which are ready to come off as the new, fresh skin emerges below.

Anti-aging

Anti-aging properties in Epsom Salt from the hydrated magnesium and sulfate help to lessen the aging effect of oxidation and environmental pollution. Make this a great way to make your own facial deep cleanse and anti-wrinkle cream too. Just leave the facial cleanser and Epsom Salt mix you made above on your face for ten minutes or more before you wipe it off with the cool damp cloth.

<u>Body cleansing</u>

Shower Sock

For those hit and run moments when a bath would be nice but a shower is more practical just grab a couple of handfuls of Epsom Salt and rub them over your body. Let the shower sluice away the grains of salt and leave your skin smooth and soft.

If you have an old white sock you can fill it with Epsom Salt and tie the top with a pretty piece of ribbon to secure the salt. Keep this in your shower and use it as a body wipe to help detox, exfoliate and smooth your body. Once the salt has dissolved the sock can be refilled again.

Milk Baths

Epsom Salt is so good for bathing in for health reasons that it makes sense to incorporate them into your routine beauty bathing too. Milk baths are popular because they moisturize your skin and add a bit of a luxury to bathtime. Before you get into the bath:

1. Add together half a cup of powdered milk (personally I love almond milk as it smells wonderful) and half a cup of Epsom Salt.
2. Drop in three drops of any essential oil of your choice.
3. Rose essential oil is a particularly sweet oil to use for this – but if you have a favorite such as ylang-ylang use that.
4. The oil is just to make the occasion into a deluxe experience!

5. Add a splash of water. Just enough to make a paste so be sure to add a tablespoon at a time so you can control the consistency.

6. Once your paste is made, rub it onto the dry skin areas on your body.

7. Favorite areas are elbows and feet but often dry scaly patches can start anywhere if you have been out in the sun.

8. Give yourself a minute or two for the paste to harden on your skin then pop into the bath and soak.

9. If there is any extra paste in the bowl tip it into the bath too.

Give yourself at least 20 minutes of luxuriating time and then wipe off any remaining paste with the facecloth.

Get out of the bath and enjoy the sensation of softness and perfume surrounding you.

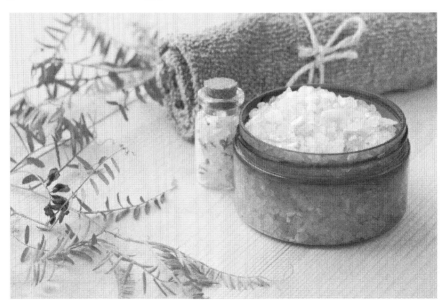

Epsom Salt Bath Bombs

Before you start, assemble the following ingredients:

Dry Ingredients

- 1 cup Baking Soda
- Half cup Citric acid powder
- Half cup Epsom Salt

Wet ingredients

- 2 teaspoons Olive oil
- 2 teaspoons Witch Hazel
- 1 teaspoon Vanilla essence
- Essential oil of your choice such as citrus, bergamot …
- Dried herb of your choice such as ginger powder
- Silicon baking moulds or muffin pans.
- Bowl to mix in
- Wooden spoon

Instructions:

1. Mix together the dry ingredients and put aside.
2. Mix together the wet ingredients and stir them well.
3. Quickly add the dry and the wet ingredients together and mix well using a spoon or your hands.
4. The mixture should stick together like a pastry dough with no crumbling.
5. Add a little water or more witch hazel if it is still a bit dry.
6. Then quickly roll into balls and push into the silicon molds or greased muffin pans. Press each one in firmly and cover.
7. Leave to dry and if you peep under the cover from time to time and notice that they are expanding this is right.

8. Just gently push them down again to stop them from expanding too much.
9. After they are dry (a day or two) put them in an airtight container and store.

These bombs last up to a year and are great presents too.

Masks and Moisturizing

Getting rid of acne – and removing blackheads – can be done by adding a teaspoon of Epsom salts to 3 drops of iodine and mixing into a half cup of hot water. Using a cotton swab wipe over the infected or blocked pores. Leave for a couple of minutes then again sluice off with lukewarm water.

For chronic acne another home remedy using Epson Salt is to whip up one egg white until it forms stiff peaks, add in a teaspoon of aloe vera, a teaspoon of Epsom Salt, a mashed up ripe tomato and a half teaspoon of Vit B5 powder then drip in one or two drops of an essential oil of your choice. Thyme or Lavender are both good as they are antibiotic and soothing. Smooth into face or areas where acne is severe and wait for a quarter of an hour before rinsing off. Doing this regularly can have a wonderful effect on the infected areas.

Petroleum Jelly (a quarter of a cup) added to two cups of Epsom Salt makes another excellent mask and a deep penetrating moisturizer. Great for the hardened skin on the soles of your feet or calluses on your hands. Also you can use this as a gentle gloss for your lips when they become chapped by winter wind and cold.

Bentonite clay is another excellent companion for Epsom Salt when you want to make a mask. Mixed together they can be used for facial masks or body masks.

For a body mask use:

- Half a cup of Bentonite Clay powder (Ebay is a good source)
- Half a cup Epsom Salt
- A drop of the essential oil of your choice.

Instructions:

1. Pour the Epsom Salt into the bath water and add the drop of essential oil.
2. Put a small amount of water in the cup with the Clay and make up a stiff paste.
3. Mix well using a wooden spoon (not metal) so that the lumps work themselves out.
4. Smear the paste on your body and give yourself another 5 minutes of air drying the paste before climbing into the Epsom Salt and essential oil bath.
5. Soak for at least 20 minutes.
6. Use the facecloth for removing any last bits of clay as you get out of the bath.
7. As you will know from the Health Section this is a powerful combination as the Bentonite Clay works to pull out toxins from the body and the Epsom Salt also detoxifies the body and gently releases the sulfate and magnesium to be absorbed through the skin.
8. Bear in mind that the warmer you have the water the stronger the detox will be and this means that you will gain the most benefit by resting and relaxing on the bed afterwards.

Hair Care

Make a hairspray

Tired of having your eyes water and sneezing your head off after a spray of bought 'hair product'? Making your own with Epsom Salt is a great, and very economical, option.

- 3 tablespoons Epsom salt
- Half a teaspoon pink sea salt or Himalayan Salt
- 1 teaspoon Aloe Vera gel
- 2 drops of essential oil, choosing one of your favorite scents
- 1 cup of hot tea as the base. Use Chamomile for light hair and Black, everyday tea for dark hair.
- I spray bottle which can be bought from many chemists

Instructions:
1. Add all ingredients to the bottle and shake well until the Salts are dissolved.
2. Store this in your fridge between uses and it will last up to four months.

Remove hairspray

On the other hand sometimes you can have a buildup of hair spray on your hair which makes it looks dull. In this case you can use your Epsom Salt again to come to the rescue.

- 2 liters water
- Half cup lemon juice
- Half cup Epsom Salt.

Instructions:
1. Mix together and leave overnight.

2. The next day pour the mixture on your dry hair before washing it.
3. Wrap an old towel around your head and do something else for 20 minutes.
4. After this wash your hair as normal and enjoy how soft, refreshed and shiny it has become.

Volumize hair

There are some days when your hair just seems to be lank. Or maybe you have long fine hair that lies in smooth straight sheets, but you want some volume in it when you go out. Epsom Salt steps into the breach again:

Take:
- Half a cup of your best deep hair conditioner
- Half a cup of Epsom Salt

Instructions:
1. Stir these together and gently warm in a pan.
2. Then take the warmed mixture and work it into your dry hair.
3. Using an old towel wrap this around your treated hair and wait for twenty minutes. Rinse your hair thoroughly and style as usual.

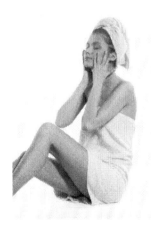

Hair Protection

If you are having some pampering time at your local beauty spa or swimming baths Epsom Salt can protect your hair when it is in the harsher environment of the steam room, sauna or chlorinated pool. Using the same recipe as above put the warmed and combined mixture in a jar and take it to the Spa. Enjoy a swim then when you come out of the pool coat your hair with the mixture and pull on a hair turban or wrap a towel around your head and then go into the steam or heat rooms. Twenty minutes or more to let the Salt do its magic and then rinse off in the shower. Comb through and style.

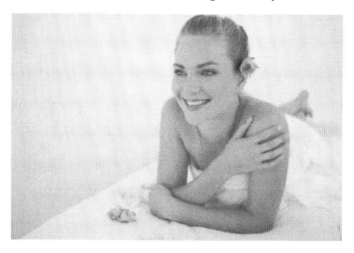

It also works well if you enjoy all the spa treatment rooms and then wash your hair, apply the mix, wrap your towel around your head and go through to the resting lounge. A browse through a magazine will take up about twenty minutes and then a quick rinse off in the shower again before you style your hair and get dressed. It is particularly useful if you use a hair dryer for styling your hair which can encourage split ends. The Epsom Salt mix strengthens your hair beautifully.

Chapter 6:
Epsom Salt in Your Home

Household Uses of Epsom Salt

The introduction of hydrated Magnesium Sulphate to the household tasks makes life easier – and cheaper. Epsom Salt is a cleanser and antiseptic solution and also works well with Hydrogen Peroxide which is a bleach. The two combined make for a powerful cleaner for many areas that get grimy but are difficult to clean.

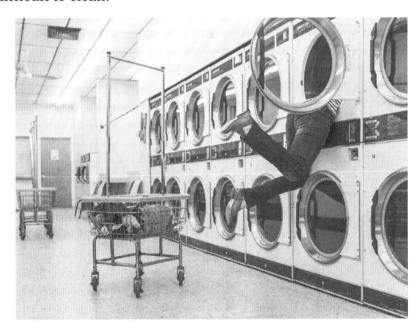

Bathroom

Wonderful for tiles and the grouting in between them. Use a toothbrush to work it in, leave for five minutes then sluice off. Polish with a clean dry cloth. Use I cup Epsom Salt to 1 cup dishwashing liquid and mix together well.

41

Kitchen

Using the same mix as above use around taps where an accumulation of limescale can form. Toothbrush helps to work the mix in and also acts as a slight abrasive on the lime scale, roughening it so the Epsom Salt can work into a bigger surface.

Mix half cup Epsom Salt with a quarter cup of baby oil. Add a couple of drops of a favorite essential oil too. Mix well by shaking in a jar or old shampoo bottle. Use as a hand wash to both clean and moisturize hands after working at the sink.

That hardened crust of burnt food in your pans and dishes will come right off with the help of a quarter of a tablespoon of Epsom salt and mix with the warm water you run in to soften the crust. Leave it to soak and do its work before scrubbing with a scourer and rinsing off. The crust will come off easily with this method.

Scullery/Laundry

Fill up your washing machine with hot water and throw in 3 cups of Epsom salt. Set the machine to run the 'quick' or 'economy' wash cycle. This will help to lift the detergent build up in the metal parts of the machine and clean it thoroughly.

Garage

If you have made up a solution of Epsom Salt and water for your first aid box as we looked at in the last chapter, make a double quantity and fill up another bottle for the garage too. Unbeatable for getting batteries going again when they have 'died' overnight. Just dampen the contacts and try again. Sometimes making a paste of Epsom Salt and water and putting the paste on the contact points works well too. It all depends on what you have to hand.

Front windows

It's Christmas time and you want to make pretty patterns on your windows to recreate a visit from Jack Frost. Using a bowl add 1 cup Epsom Salt to half a cup of water and stir in 3 tablespoons of dishwasher liquid.

Use a sponge to dab on the windows. As it dries the salt creates the frosting. It can easily be wiped off with a warm damp cloth later.

Chapter 7:
Epsom Salt in your Garden

We already have the emergency box of Epsom salt in the garage for help with a variety of mishaps as we saw in the earlier sections. Now we make sure we have plenty of it in the potting shed – or garage – wherever you keep your garden equipment.

Epsom Salt has so many uses in the garden – fertilizer, insecticide, rescue remedy for poorly plants... Look through the following to see where you can use this plentiful and cheap powder to make your garden grow.

Fertilizer

To help new plants which you are just introducing to the garden settle in, make sure to add two or three handfuls of Epsom salt to the earth you have dug out of the hole where you will plant them. As you settle the plant into its new home pack the salted soil around the roots and stem to nourish the plant as it grows.

Use as fertilizer to help your existing plants

It is easy to deplete the ground's stock of essential elements with over planting, or by having the misfortune to live in a place where the topsoil is poor. The natural minerals needed by growing plants, such as potassium, nitrogen and phosphorus all work more effectively if they are mixed with the hydrated Magnesium Sulphate in Epsom Salt. This is especially so if you have a lot of soaking rain which dilutes the mineral all the time. Once a week go out with a bucketful of Salts and scatter a handful on your most prized flowers, houseplants and vegetables.

Grass

On an even larger scale Epsom Salt is good for the lawn to encourage new, strong and vigorous growth. Take a gallon of water and add half a cup of Epsom Salt then spray the garden with this solution. The magnesium really helps to make the green more vivid since it supports the chlorophyll production.

Flowers and Vegetables

The Salt promotes growth in two ways as it tends to make blooms or vegetables bigger and to produce more flowers/fruit or vegetables. When you are planting new flowering plants or vegetables keep scattering in Epsom salts as you plant or sow. Then keep up a weekly feed of a handful of Salt as they begin to grow. You will soon be rewarded. The most famous Epsom Salt success was a winning Pumpkin that weighed in at just over 200Kgs. A monster!

Enhance flavor in Fruit and vegetables

Epsom salt improves the flavor as well as the size and amount of your fruit and vegetables. It is particularly effective on peppers and tomatoes but any plant in your vegetable garden will benefit. Do not be afraid to use plenty of the Salt as you fertilize in this area of your garden, they can easily take three of four times as much Epsom salt as the flower garden.

Herbicide

As well as being a fertilizer for the plants you want to nurture and grow Epsom Salt can be used as a weedkiller. Mix a litre of water with 2 tablespoons of Epsom Salt and 1 tablespoon of ordinary dishing washing liquid. Shake this up then spray it on the weeds you want to get rid of and you will find that the weeds die back but the magnesium and sulphate sink into the ground leaving the soil ready for you to plant something more suitable.

Rescue Remedy for Curling Leaves

Citrus leaves can suddenly turn very curly, as can some other bushes, and this is usually a sign of lack of magnesium and is also helped by several handfuls of Epsom Salt to get the healing underway then regular handfuls weekly thereafter. Don't forget that 'skin' has the ability to absorb nutrients too and the same goes for leaves. It is possible to add Epsom Salt to your sprayer and coat the curly leaves with the solution of 1 cup Salt to 1 liter water. Make sure the salt is well dissolved first. Preferably do both the spraying and the feeding of the soil to help the curly leaves. Water the dry Salt in well so it soaks to the roots unless you know it will rain soon.

Before you plant your seedlings or new bushes soak the roots in Epsom Salt solution of half a cup of Salt to one gallon of water.

Leave overnight then plant. Let the root ball become saturated with the Salt water.

Not only roses benefit from a weekly scattering of Epsom Salts. Rhododendron and Azaleas tend to turn yellow when the sulfate level of the soil gets too low. One tablespoon over the root area every month helps with this. Water in well.

Other plants that do well with a drenching of Epsom Salt solution when they turn yellow are ferns, cycads, bougainvillea and gardenia. With their heavy flowering these last two strip the ground of magnesium so scattering half a cupful over the ground around them can replenish the lost minerals. Large leaved plants benefit from spraying with a solution of Epsom Salt made from a tablespoon of Salt to one gallon of water.

As you move into a property and start working the garden there are often old tree stumps that have been left to rot in the ground but cling tenaciously to life with parts dead and other parts very weak. Because Epsom Salt absorbs water so well it works to drill a series of holes in the trunk and pack Epsom Salt into them. Also scatter the Salt over any old exposed roots. As the moisture is pulled out of the old stump it will become weaker and weaker and after several applications of the Salt you can uproot the old stump and start your own new project at last.

Insecticide

Slugs hate Epsom salt! So do most plant pests, so although I wouldn't stop doing your companion planting and using other natural means of pest control, spraying with Epsom salt is another addition to the arsenal against these little pests. Slugs are different! They don't like to slide over the crystals of Magnesium Sulfate so will steer clear of the areas which are regularly dusted with Epsom salt. It doesn't kill them in the way that ordinary salt does, but it does encourage them to go elsewhere!

BONUS CHAPTER

Aromatherapy Recipes & Essential Oil Blends for Your Epsom Salt Baths

The following aromatherapy recipes can be mixed with Epsom salt to enhance your Epsom salt relaxation baths! You can also use them on your own to create your holistic oils. These are fantastic for self-massage after your Epsom salt bath experience.

EO in the recipes means= essential oil

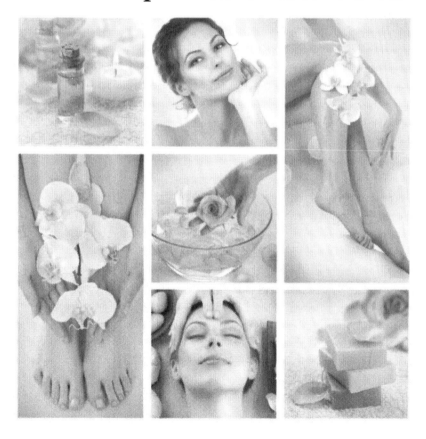

Sweet Dreams-Fight Insomnia

Blend:

- 2 tablespoons of coconut oil or olive oil (sesame oil works great too)
- 2 drops of verbena EO +
- 2 drops of lavender (or lavandin) EO +
- 2 drops of mandarin EO +

Add to your Epsom salt bath or use for self-massage.

Amazing Energy!

Sick and tired of feeling sick and tired?

Try this recipe!

Blend:

- 1 tablespoon of coconut oil
- 2 drops of Camomila Noble EO+
- 2 drops of Mandarine EO+
- 2 drops of Rosemary EO

Add to your Epsom salt bath or use for self-massage.

You can also apply via neck and head massage. It will be extremely invigorating. Moreover, head massage is a great natural hair treatment. Rosemary essential oil can help you grow strong healthy hair and prevent hair loss. It's also very energizing!

Healing Blend

Blend:

- 1 tablespoon of coconut oil or other roil (olive, sesame, almond) you like
- 2 drops of verbena EO+
- 2 drops of ylang ylang EO

Add to your Epsom salt bath or use for self-massage.

Easy Anti-Flu Mix

Blend:

- 2 tablespoons of coconut oil or other natural oil of your choice
- 2 drops of Moroccan thyme EO+
- 2 drops of eucalyptus Citriodora EO
- 2 drops of tea tree EO

Add to your Epsom salt bath or use for self-massage.

Lymphatic Help Blend

If you suffer from varicose veins, fluid retention as well as cellulite this recipe will help you rejuvenate your legs. Try to soak in an Epsom salt bath first, or add Epsom salt to your peeling. Then, prepare this aromatherapy blend for leg massage.

You can also add the following mix to your regular Epsom salt bath and take advantage of its relaxing properties, enjoy!

Blend:

- 2 tablespoons coconut oil
- 2 drops of grapefruit EO+
- 2 drops of peppermint EO+
- 2 drops of juniper EO+
- 2 drops of geranium EO

For a massage:

Massage this blend gently into your legs, start from the feet and ankles and move up so as to stimulate venous circulation.

Grapefruit, juniper and geranium work as a natural lymphatic drainage and mint gives an instant sensation of coolness and energy. Great for swollen and tired legs after a hard day at work.

Headache Remover

Blend:

- 2 tablespoons of coconut oil or other holistic oil of your choice
- 2 drops of lavandin+
- 2 drops of verbena +
- 2 drops of mint EO

Add to your Epsom salt bath or use for self-massage.

Massage instructions:

Massage forehead and temples gently and massage the neck. You can also do a scalp massage for better results, but normally a simple forehead massage (make sure you squeeze your eyebrows) will make the pain go away in less than 5 minutes.

Natural Coffee for Your Soul!

This holistic recipe will help you wake up and restore your energy levels. You can also use it for meditation, as it will help you keep centered.

Blend:

- 1 tablespoon of coconut oil
- 2 drops of citronella EO+
- 1 drop of cinnamon EO+
- 1 drops of bergamot EO+
- 1 drop of ylang ylang

Add to your Epsom salt bath or use for self-massage.

Massage instructions:

1. Massage your neck, chest, and shoulders. Head massage with oils can be extremely energizing too.
2. You will find the balance between citric scents like citronella and bergamot spiced up by floral ylang ylang fragrance and cinnamon mystery.
3. Bergamot is also a great anti-anxiety remedy as my next recipe explains.
4. Remember- no sunbathing after this massage! Citric oils are photo-toxic.

No More Anxiety!

If you feel like anxiety is knocking on your door make sure you take a few deep breaths and confide in aromatherapy and Epsom salt combo.

With this blend you can take a holistic approach and get to the root of the problem.

This is so much better than standard anti-anxiety pills that only make us sick and tired (and very often fat).

You already know that Epsom salt bath is a great source of magnesium (a mineral you need to fight stress). If you combine it with essential oils, you will give yourself an amazing mix of all natural ingredients to fight anxiety.

Blend:

- 2 tablespoons of coconut oil
- 2 drops of bergamot+
- 2 drops of verbena+
- 2 drops of basil (refrain from using this oil if you are suffering from clinical depression).

Add to your Epsom salt bath or use for self-massage.

Massage Instructions:

You can do a full body massage.

Concentrate on your feet and solar plexus.

Breathe in and out in a conscious way.

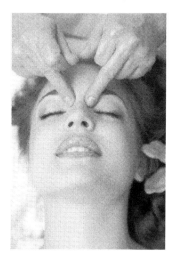

For Athletes

Blend:

- 2 tablespoons of coconut oil or other natural oil of your choice
- 2 drops of clove EO
- 2 drops of basil EO+
- 2 drops of rosemary EO

Add to your Epsom salt bath or use for self-massage. (focus on sore areas)

Easy Relax Sweet Mix

Blend:

- 2 tablespoons of coconut oil or other oil of your choice
- 2 drops of mandarin EO+
- 2 drop of mint EO+
- 2 drops of juniper EO+

Add to your Epsom salt bath or use for self-massage.

AROMATHERAPY PRECAUTIONS

Aromatherapy General Precautions

Aromatherapy is a very safe and easy therapy to use, but keep in mind that there are certain precautions:

- Remember to wash your hands after applying aromatherapy massage;

- Do not apply the essential oils in their pure form as they may cause an allergic reaction. Instead, use blends that contain 2-5% essential oils diluted in good-quality cold-pressed oil;

-After using citrus oils, like for example lemon, verbena, bergamot, orange etc. avoid direct sun exposure, even up to 8 hours after the treatment

- Do not apply oils after surgery (unless you have consulted with a doctor) or on open wounds or rashes of unknown origin;

- Do not use the oils after chemotherapy (unless suggested by a doctor);

- Keep the oils away from the eyes and mucus membranes;

- Use the oils only topically, do not ingest them (unless you are working with a certified scientific aromatherapist)

- Avoid rosemary, thyme, Spanish and common sage, fennel and hyssop if you suffer from high blood pressure;

- Do not apply the treatments described in this book on babies or infants. It doesn't mean that aromatherapy can never be used on babies and infants, but extremely low concentrations should be used. Always consult with a medical or naturopathy doctor first;

- After an aromatherapy massage always remember to wash your hands;

- Make sure that you research the brand, read safety instructions for each individual oil you buy/use and check the expiration date;

- Store your blends in dark glass bottles, preferably in a cool, dry and dark place and remember to use within a maximum of one month after mixing.

BONUS CHAPTER 2

How to Combine Epsom Salt with Mindfulness Meditation

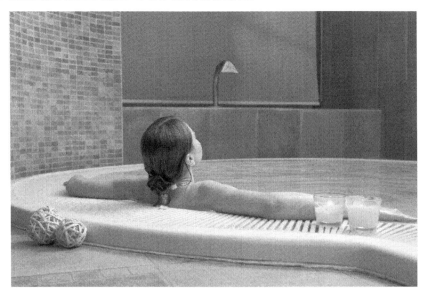

Here is something to think about and practice while enjoying your Epsom salt bath...Meditation is not only about spending hours on meditation cushions, you can practice it wherever you want, and it's always better if you feel relaxed (Epsom salt bath with essential oils is great for that).

Recent decades have seen a groundswell of research into the benefits of mindfulness meditation. Mindfulness's many benefits are now a part of general public knowledge and accepted scientific fact. Among these benefits are:

- deeper concentration and less tendency to distraction
- the ability to focus on the present moment
- an increase in nonjudgmental awareness
- the ability to see your emotions objectively

- letting go of outdated identities
- a general increase in positive emotions

How to practice mindfulness meditation

Practicing mindfulness meditation is quite simple and does not require a lot of preparation or training. Anyone can get into it. All you have to do is make a little time. *Learning how* to do the practice *is* the practice.

To begin with, set aside five to ten minutes of your day, every day. Find a quiet place to sit- a nice warm bath is great for that. Whatever works for you.

Your eyes can be open or closed; it's up to you. You may find that closing your eyes helps keep you from distraction, at least in the beginning.

The basic practice of sitting meditation is just to place your mind on the breath. *Mindfulness* in this context means being mindful of the breath, just following it as it moves in and out. When thoughts and sensations arise, you notice them and simply return your attention to the breath. It does not really matter what kind of thoughts or feelings come up. They could be boring thoughts about what you need to get from the store, or they could be mean, angry, happy, funny, creative, passionate—whatever.

Whatever comes up, just mentally label it *thinking* and return your attention to the breath. That's the nonjudgmental awareness we talked about earlier—whatever comes up, don't try to decide whether it's good or bad, don't accept or reject it. Just gently say to yourself, *Thinking*, and gently redirect your attention to the breath.

As you follow the breath in and out, you want to pay attention to the sensation of the breath—the feeling of the cool in-breath on your nostrils, and the warmth of the out-breath, the rise and fall of your lungs as you breathe in and out, whether the breath is long or short, shallow or deep, hard or gentle, and so on. In general, when meditating on the breath, you don't try to change the quality of the breath, but just let your lungs breathe however is most natural at any given time, and watch that.

Breathing is an effortless, autonomic function of the body, so we normally don't pay any attention to it. It just goes on in the background, all the time. In the practice of mindfulness, however, we don't take the breath for granted. Instead, we learn to appreciate the breath in its simplicity and variation. We develop a sense of wonder at something so simple and so necessary—taking in lungful of healthful, life-giving oxygen, which are delivered to the different organs of our body by the circulation of our blood. If we can learn to love and appreciate the simple fact of being alive, we can love ourselves.

When you begin meditating, it may seem that your discursive thoughts, the so-called "monkey mind," have only increased. Actually, nothing has increased; you just never noticed how active your mind is. Just stick with the practice of remaining mindful of the breath. Slowly, the speed of your thoughts will decrease. You will begin to notice and enjoy the vivid richness of the direct, sensory quality of your experience. This is the beginning of coming in touch with a quality of yourself that is fundamentally awake. It is the discovery of an innate source of goodness deep within your being.

Making friends with yourself

By breathing your awareness to the breath and learning to appreciate the simplicity of the present moment, you develop a sense of love for yourself that is not based on stories that you tell yourself, your wishes, likes and dislikes, who you tell yourself you want to be, negative thoughts, and so on. Instead, this newfound self-love is based on a direct, honest relationship to your own mind. This relationship is what has been called *making friends with yourself*.

The very act of meditation is an act of kindness to yourself. By setting aside time to rest and watch the breath, you are demonstrating a willingness and a commitment to sit with yourself quietly and gently. That is an act of compassion, a declaration of unconditional friendship to yourself and a willingness to get to know your own mind and heart more deeply.

It may sound strange to hear, but most of us do not really know ourselves that well. That's because we never take the time to get to know ourselves. So it's important to take that time, to slow down and rest. In this state of rest, we become more familiar with our own thoughts and feelings. Through the process of making friends with ourselves in meditation, we equip ourselves with self-love and self-compassion. Thus we can forgive ourselves when we make mistakes, or offer ourselves gentle encouragement and advice when we feel overwhelmed or anxious. This becomes a safeguard against the pessimism that attacks our motivation.

Deeper Concentration

It's easy to see how improving your concentration can increase your motivation to achieve your goals. In our daily lives, we're assailed from all sides by distractions and events vying for our attention. Meditation helps keep us on track by reducing the noise inside our heads. With more mindfulness, we will feel empowered to work towards our goals without going off track.

By bringing us into the present moment, mindfulness meditation helps induce a creative state of awareness psychologists call *flow*. Flow is full absorption in an activity with energetic focus and enjoyment. Research shows that mindfulness increases flow, focus, sharp thinking, self-control, and even the ability to meet deadlines.

Focus on the present moment

It's often helpful to clarify what you want for the future. If you know your desired outcome, that positive vision of the future can give you the energy that spurs you along on your journey to health and wellness you deserve.

Stress

A big part of stress is a physiological response in the body that psychologists call "fight or flight" mode. Stress is basically a response to something that your body and brain experience as a threat. So your heart rate increases, your muscles tense up, your breathing accelerates, blood pressure goes up, your digestive system is inhibited.

None of this is a problem if you're staring down a predator in the jungle. In fact, it's a good thing, because it gets you ready to either fight for your life, or run away very fast. And, in the wilderness, you'll need to do one of those things if you hope to live.

But in our hectic modern lives, it's often the case that what our brain experiences as a threat does not go away. So we stay in fight-or-flight for days, months, years. We can't sleep properly, often we don't feel like eating, and we're generally just miserable. Eventually it takes a big toll on our health and can lead to a number of diseases.

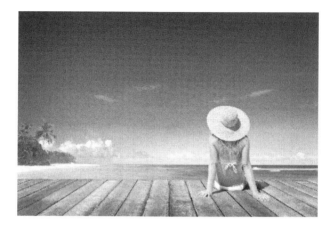

The good news is that meditation just by itself is shown to reduce stress very effectively. In addition to that, however, there are a few things you can do to bring your stress levels down. The most important thing to do is find ways to rest. Even if you are very busy, take some *me* time to just relax.

By "resting" I don't just mean sleeping, although that's important, too. I mean doing things that you find intrinsically enjoyable—that you don't have to force yourself to do, because you *want* to do them. That can be enjoying a tasty meal, talking a long walk in the afternoon, going for a swim, spending time with loved ones. Exercise is an excellent method for lowering stress, as is relaxing with friends and family.

The basic idea is that, since your brain thinks you are in danger, you need to do things that make the brain feel safe. You don't have to force your stress levels down. Just engage in some restful, enjoyable activity, and the stress will go down all by itself.

Healing from the inside out!

****

So....now you have reached the end of the fascinating journey into the world of Epsom Salt. Can you believe just how many uses it has? I hope by now you have been persuaded to add Epsom Salt to your shopping list and that you have already had your first Salt Spa in your very own bathroom. Whatever use you decide to put Epsom Salt to I hope you enjoy the experience and jeep this book to hand to check on quantities to use or to check for ideas.

Wishing you good health and a happy home!

Let's connect:

www.facebook.com/HolisticWellnessBooks

www.twitter.com/Wellness_Books

Book 2

Apple Cider Vinegar

The Miraculous Natural Remedy!

Holistic Solutions & Proven Healing *Recipes*

for

Health, Beauty and Home!

by Elena Garcia

www.facebook.com/HolisticWellnessBooks

From the Author

Thank You for taking an interest in my book. It really means a lot to me. In appreciation, I would like to offer you a free complimentary PDF eBook + access to our health and wellness newsletter.

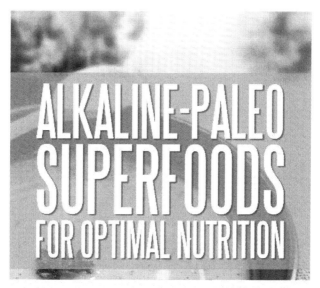

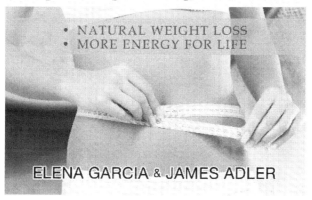

Download link:

www.holisticwellnessbooks.com/bonus

Apple Cider Vinegar- Introduction

Apple Cider Vinegar is one of those items that your home and kitchen would just not be complete without. It has so many uses that after reading this book you would wonder why you never tried it before. Apple Cider Vinegar is one of, if not the most popular vinegar within the natural health industry and its extensive benefits are a clear indication of why this is so. It is available in both an organic variety and a non-organic variety and the quality of the available products will differ, however they all have the same uses and benefits; obviously organic would be the best choice, but not necessarily the most cost-effective.

Apple Cider Vinegar is made in a two step process, much like most vinegar, first the apples are crushed, and they are then exposed to yeast which ferments the natural sugars within the apples causing a production of alcohol. Bacteria are then added to the now alcoholic solution, which further ferments it turning it into acetic acid, which is the main active compound in all vinegars. The organic, unfiltered varieties also contain proteins and enzymes that give the vinegar a murky appearance, thus the less clear the appearance of the vinegar, the more organic and less filtered it will be. The unfiltered varieties are also known to contain what is referred to as the "mother strand" which is what gives the vinegar a cob-web-like appearance. The mother of vinegar is composed of a form of cellulose and acetic acid bacteria which forms as a result of the fermenting of alcoholic liquids; therefore it would form during the process of adding bacteria to the crushed apple and yeast base that begins the making of Apple Cider Vinegar.

Apple Cider Vinegar is very low in calories; containing only three calories per tablespoon (15ml). Apple Cider Vinegar doesn't boast a decent content of vitamins and minerals, however it does contain a small amount of potassium, which is incredibly important for muscle recovery and many other functions within the body. Thus, as far as nutrition is concerned, Apple Cider Vinegar doesn't come to the party, however since it is known for, and celebrated, for so many other reasons it could be argued that it is still an ingredient that would be a necessity to any shopping list.

This book aims to show and enlighten you to all of the uses and benefits of Apple Cider Vinegar in terms of health and wellness, treating ailments, home use, beauty use and an extra section that includes recipe ideas that will help you further incorporate Apple Cider Vinegar into your daily routine. The side-effects and precautions of using Apple Cider Vinegar will also be explored and noted within its own chapter in order to make sure that you will be using and incorporating this vinegar into your regular routine without putting yourself at any risk or creating any harm to your health or body, so it will be important to take note of the chapter that deals with this related topic.

Chapter One:
Health Benefits and Uses of Apple Cider Vinegar

Apple cider vinegar has a number of uses in terms of health, healing and remedies. This chapter will explore all of these benefits and uses and aims to enlighten you to this incredibly useful and cost effective source of natural healing. It is important to note that the chapter to follow will look at the possible side-effects and precautions of using apple cider vinegar as a treatment and remedy for health issues and preventative measures, therefore it is suggested that one reads both chapters before beginning the use of apple cider vinegar for such purposes.

Apple Cider Vinegar for Tummy Trouble and Digestive Concerns:

If you are suffering from diarrhea that is caused by a bacterial infection, the natural antibiotic and anti-bacterial properties of apple cider vinegar will make this home remedy a great option when looking to treat the symptoms of such and infection without the use of an over the counter chemical based drug. Apple cider vinegar is also known to help ease the spasms and stomach cramps that generally come with such an infection, this is a result of the high pectin content that apple cider vinegar is known to contain. To use apple cider vinegar as a remedy in this instance you would mix one tablespoon (15ml) of apple cider vinegar into one cup (250ml) of water or clear apple juice; this mixture should be sipped slowly so as not to upset the stomach an further.

Apple Cider Vinegar to Help Ease and Cure Hiccups:

Hiccups can be triggered by a number of things such as drinking alcohol, smoking, having a bloated stomach, eating too fast or eating foods that are too spicy, consuming fizzy drinks or emotions such as stress, fear or excitement. Hiccups are a result of an irritation and upset to the natural movement of the diaphragm, causing it to suck in air as it closes. This air causes the diaphragm to pull down with a jerk causing air to be sucked into the throat; the actual hiccup happens when this air rushes back up the esophagus and hits into the vocal chords. To use apple cider vinegar as remedy for hiccups take one tablespoon (15ml) of neat apple cider vinegar as you would drink cough mixture. The apple cider vinegar works in this instance because its high acetic acid content will overstimulate the throat resulting in the relaxing of the nerves within the throat that are causing the spasms that are resulting in the hiccup motion.

Apple Cider Vinegar to Sooth a Sore Throat:

A sore throat can be a result of a number of things, but the most common cause is generally a post nasal drip that can be the result of a mild sinus infection or head cold. Bacteria containing mucus drips down the back of the throat cavity causing the throat to become inflamed and painful. The anti-bacterial and antibiotic properties of apple cider vinegar make it a very useful natural home remedy for this particular health concern. To use apple cider vinegar to treat a sore throat mix ¼ cup (60ml) apple cider vinegar into ¼ cup (60ml) warm water and gargle with this solution on an hourly basis until you no longer feel that scratchy pain when swallowing. If symptoms persist and you still have a sore throat after forty eight hours of using this home remedy, it is then recommended that you consult with your doctor as you may have a more severe infection that possibly requires a harsher treatment.

Apple Cider Vinegar to Lower Blood Cholesterol:

Unfortunately there is not a lot of backing evidence and research into the theory that apple cider vinegar can indeed lower blood cholesterol. However there have been studies conducted that revealed a noted drop in the blood cholesterol levels of people who participated in the study; these participants consumed one tablespoon (15ml) of apple cider vinegar per day over the course of the study. It must be noted that blood cholesterol levels are linked to many chronic diseases and there is no single cure for it; the best way to create and maintain a healthy blood cholesterol level is by making sure that you are living a healthy, well-balance lifestyle that includes a balanced diet and sufficient exercise. It is recommended that if you have a family history of high blood cholesterol you should have your levels checked at least every one to two years and the most accurate form of testing is a fasting blood test. If you predict that you may have, or you know that you do have, high blood cholesterol levels then it is highly recommended that you consult with your physician regarding this; also it is not recommended that you pursue treatment of this concern using apple cider vinegar without consulting with your physician first.

Apple Cider Vinegar to Prevent Indigestion:

Since no two human beings are completely the same; there are certain foods and food combinations that either agree or disagree with one's digestive system. There are also those special occasions such as weddings or birthday parties where we all have the tendency to over-indulge in foods that we wouldn't normally eat on a regular basis. These could be foods that are higher in salt, fat and sugar than those that we would normally consume. Some people find the consumption of very spicy food tasty, but it can cause an irritation to their digestive systems. Everyone has their own little niggle when it comes to these things. Apple cider vinegar is a great preventative measure in such instances. To use apple cider vinegar as preemptive and preventative measure when you know or suspect that you will be over indulging in foods that may cause you to be sorry a few hours afterward mix one teaspoon (5ml) of apple cider vinegar and one teaspoon (5ml) of natural pure honey into one cup (250ml) of warm water and drink this solution half an hour before your over-indulgent meal.

Apple Cider Vinegar to Clear a Stuffy Nose:

Nasal congestion and a stuffy nose that usually comes as a side-effect of the common head cold virus is caused by a bacterial infection within the nasal and sinus cavity. Such viral infections are known to hit even the healthiest of people during the change of seasons when there are a number of viral spores floating around in the air all around us. Nasal congestion and stuffy nose can be incredibly uncomfortable and irritating; it can also lead to other concerns for example, a blocked nose will lead to one breathing through their mouth since the nasal cavity does not a have free-flowing source of air. Breathing through the mouth for an extended period of time most often leads to a dry and scratchy throat which will create further discomfort. Due to apple cider vinegar's anti-bacterial and antibiotic properties as well as its high acetic acid content, together with the potassium that is is known to contain; it will help thin the mucus that is generally the cause of the nasal congestion that one would be experiencing in a case like this. To use apple cider vinegar as a natural home remedy for nasal congestion mix one teaspoon (5ml) of apple cider vinegar into one cup (250ml) of water and drink. This can be repeated three times a day. It is important to note that if symptoms of your head cold or virus persist for longer than three days there is the possibility that you may have a more severe strain of the common virus and it would be highly recommended that you consult with your physician in this case as you may need a harsher form of treatment.

Apple Cider Vinegar to Aid in Weight Loss:

The maintenance of a healthy weight and good looking body is something that we all strive for and are consistently concerned about. There are many natural forms of healthy weight loss and maintenance, and these are always the better option rather than chemical based drugs that claim to give you the quick fix that we all wish was possible. The truth is that there is no quick fix to weight loss and maintenance and that this is only achieved through a well balanced healthy lifestyle that focuses on a balanced diet and exercise regime. However there are many natural forms of help that we can call upon in order to move the process along. Apple cider vinegar helps in this instance due to its high acetic acid content which is known to suppress appetite, boost metabolism, and reduce water retention which is a common cause of a higher number on the scale. Some scientists believe that apple cider vinegar can help the body and the digestive system in the breaking down of starch and carbohydrates, allowing them to move through your system more easily and to be absorbed in a more efficient way that does not lead to fat gain.

Apple Cider Vinegar to Help in the Treatment and Prevention of Dandruff:

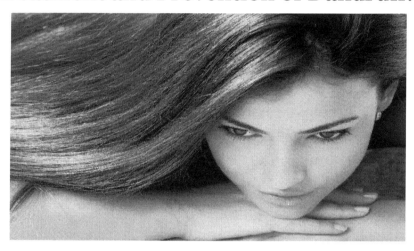

Dandruff is a common concern and many people suffer from it. The skin is the body's biggest organ and is constantly renewing and regenerating itself; as the skin renews its cells the old ones are pushed to the surface of the skin and flake off, in many people this is unnoticeable and can most likely only ever be seen on one's bath towel or face cloth. For some people this process happens at a faster rate than in others, particularly where the renewal of skin cells on the scalp are concerned. When this renewal of scalpel skin cells happens at a fast rate it results in white flakes of skin that become visible due to their accumulation in the hair, they then begin to fall to the shoulders resulting visible white flakes on your clothing; this is what is known as dandruff.

In some cases people may experience excessive flaking as a result of an underlying fungal or yeast infection. Skin conditions such as psoriasis and seborrheaic dermatitis can also lead to dandruff and excessive skin flaking.

Apple cider vinegar can help in this instance due to the fact that acidity of the vinegar changes the pH level of the skin on your scalp which will in turn make it harder for the infection-causing yeast to grow. To use apple cider vinegar as a remedy for dandruff mix ¼ cup (60ml) of apple cider vinegar with ¼ cup (60ml) of water into a spray bottle. Spray the solution generously onto your scalp before wrapping your head in a towel and allowing the solution to sit on your scalp for fifteen to twenty minutes. Wash your hair as usual and repeat this remedy twice a week.

Apple Cider Vinegar to Help Clear Acne:

In most cases severe acne is caused by an over-production of sebum by the sebaceous glands in the skin; this leads to an oilier than usual skin and can cause pimples and whiteheads, this is usually due to bacterial infection that is caused by dirt from the environment contaminating the excess sebum that is sitting on top of the skin. Very often this over-stimulation of the sebaceous glands can be induced by hormonal changes or imbalances, an irritation to the skin, or sensitivity to certain products or foods.

Apple cider vinegar can help in this instance due to its anti-bacterial and antibiotic properties which makes it a great natural and cost-effective facial toner. This is due to the malic and lactic acids that form part of the vinegar's makeup; these specific acids act as exfoliates and softeners to the skin's surface, restoring its pH balance and resulting in the reduction and treatment of red spots and their inflammation.

Apple Cider Vinegar to Boost Energy:

Intense exercise can lead to a buildup of lactic acid within the muscles of the body and this acid build up will lead to muscle stiffness and sometimes a little pain, it can also lead to both muscle and overall fatigue. This is perfectly normal and not in any way a risk, however it can become more and more uncomfortable as time goes by and that is why all professional and competing sportsmen and women all include some form of remedy for this lactic acid build-up into their daily routine.

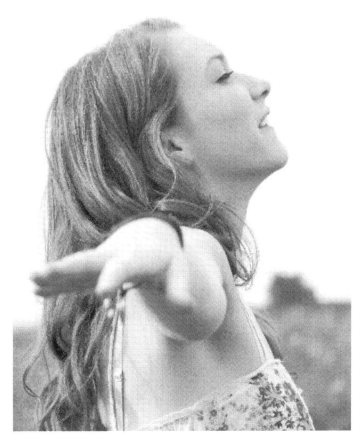

Apple cider vinegar is known to contain essential amino acids which the body uses to repair muscle fibers and boost energy levels. The potassium content in the apple cider vinegar further helps with this cause as this essential mineral is known for is potent ability to repair the normal muscle and tissue damage that comes with intense exercising; potassium is also essential in fighting both muscle and overall fatigue. To use apple cider vinegar as remedy in this instance, add one tablespoon (15ml) of apple cider vinegar to one cup (250ml) of water and drink.

Apple Cider Vinegar to Help with the Reduction of Nighttime Leg Cramps:

It's possibly safe to say that we all suffer from these excruciatingly painful leg cramps that creep up on us in the middle of the night, paralyzing your calve muscle in agonizing pain, at some point. These cramps are usually a sign that you are suffering from a deficiency in one or all of the following; sodium, magnesium or potassium. If you are sure that your body is not deficient in sodium or magnesium then the potassium content of apple cider vinegar will make it a great home remedy for this horrible, sleep disrupting cramps.

To use apple cider vinegar in this instance mix two tablespoons (30ml) of apple cider vinegar and one teaspoon (5ml) of raw organic natural honey into one cup (250ml) of warm water and drink when the cramps occur.

Apple Cider Vinegar to Help Cure Bad Breath:

Bad breath is a constant concern for all of us, and for those of us who suffer from it on a more serious level, it can be very embarrassing and can lead to one being very self-conscious. There are a number of factors that can lead to bad breath that include dental ailments, a sinus or respiratory infection, the consumption of garlic, low blood sugar levels as well as the consumption of raw onions.

Apple cider vinegar is useful as a natural remedy for bad breath due to the fact that its anti-bacterial and antibiotic properties are a great killer for bacteria that may be lurking within your mouth, causing a foul odor. To use apple cider vinegar to treat bad breath do the following; mix one teaspoon (5ml) of apple cider vinegar with one cup (250ml) water and either gargle with this solution or drink it; how you chose to use it is completely up to personal preference.

Apple Cider Vinegar to Help Whiten Teeth:

A bright, healthy and attractive smile is something that we all want, unfortunately daily lifestyle and dietary factors can result in the yellowing or staining of teeth. These factors include smoking, the drinking of coffee and tea, as well as alcohol consumption. Regular dental check-ups and visits to an oral hygienist on an annual basis are always recommended, but one can apply a home remedy in order to help the process undertaken by these healthcare professionals.

Apple cider vinegar is a cost-effective home remedy in this case and can be used to help whiten teeth. To use apple cider vinegar for this particular purpose gargle one tablespoon (15ml) of apple cider vinegar in the morning before brushing your teeth as usual.

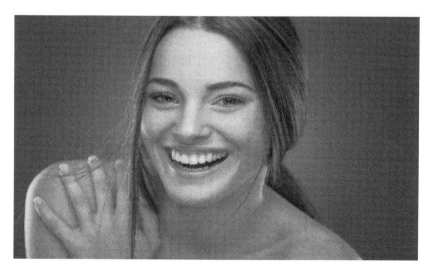

Apple Cider Vinegar to Help Fade Bruises:

Bruising is one of those unfortunate occurrences of daily life that most of us, particularly those who tend to be a little clumsier at times, simply cannot avoid. A slight bump of the knee on your desk drawer or a bump of your elbow in passing by a doorway can lead to bruising. Bruising is usually a result of a slight bleed or burst of blood vessels underneath the skin and depending on the cause can range from minor to severe in scale. There is usually an amount of inflammation that accompanies bruising.

Apple cider vinegar can be a helpful cost-effective home remedy in this instance due to its anti-inflammatory properties. To use apple cider vinegar to help fade bruises do the following; take cotton wool padding that corresponds to the size of the bruise you want to treat, soak the cotton wool in neat apple cider vinegar and lightly compress it onto the bruise. Repeat this twice a day until the bruising has faded completely.

Apple Cider Vinegar to Help Control Blood Sugar Levels:

The maintenance of balanced blood sugar levels is important in so many ways as severe drops in blood sugar can lead to all kinds of unsavory results such as headache, nausea, fatigue; and if you are watching your weight the intense hunger that usually accompanies a severe blood sugar drop can lead to the loss of self-control that results in over-indulgent eating.

If you are suffering from type two diabetes it is incredibly important to make sure that you maintain and control balanced blood sugar levels at all times. Many studies have shown a link to the home remedy of apple cider vinegar and the balancing and controlling of blood sugar levels. It is important to note that if you are aware that or you suspect that you have type two diabetes it is always highly recommended that you consult with your physician before embarking on any kind of treatment for your condition. It is also important to note that one the most effective ways of maintaining control and balance of healthy blood sugar levels is through a healthy lifestyle that includes a well-balanced diet and sufficient exercise.

To use apple cider vinegar as a means of helping to control blood sugar levels take two tablespoons (30ml) of apple cider vinegar before retiring to bed at night. One can also use apple cider vinegar as preventative measure before indulging in a high carbohydrate containing meal, that may lead to a spike in blood sugar levels; to use apple cider vinegar in this instance mix one tablespoon (15ml) of apple cider vinegar into one cup (250ml) of water and drink before your meal.

Apple Cider Vinegar to Help Clear up Yeast Infections:

A yeast infection is something that every woman will suffer from at some point in her life and is generally caused by a fluctuation in hormones, hot and sweaty environments and can also be a result of heavy sweating during exercise. Because a yeast infection is such a common medical concern it can easily be treated in a natural way.

Since apple cider vinegar has such a powerful anti-bacterial and antibiotic prevalence it is a wonderful natural remedy for treating a yeast infection. To use apple cider vinegar to treat yeast infections simply add one and a half cups (375ml) of apple cider vinegar to a warm bath and soak in the tub for approximately twenty minutes. This should be repeated once a day for the first three days of the infection.

Apple Cider Vinegar to Treat Foot and Skin Fungal Infections:

Athlete's foot is as common an infection as a yeast infection is in most people, particularly those who lead active lifestyles. Athlete's foot is commonly known as a fungal infection that affects the underside of the feet and the nail beds of the toenails; it can lead to serious discomfort and itching. Generally an anti-fungal ointment would be prescribed to treat such an infection, but these ointments are very often chemical based and can be rather harsh on the skin.

Apple cider vinegar provides a natural anti-bacterial and anti-fungal treatment for such cases. To use apple cider vinegar to treat foot and skin fungal infections you can either choose to soak the affected area in a solution of one cup (250ml) apple cider vinegar and four cups (1litre) warm water or alternatively you can apply neat apple cider vinegar directly to the affected area by soaking a cotton wool pad in the apple cider vinegar and dabbing it over the affected area.

Chapter Two: Side-Effects and Precautions to Consider When Using Apple Cider Vinegar

As with any healthcare remedy or treatment there are always significant side-effects and precautions that need to be taken into account and kept in mind at all times. Whether the treatment is natural or chemical and drug based, there are always risks involved. As mentioned in the previous chapter when using apple cider vinegar for the treatment and prevention of any medical or health problem it is always advised to seek professional medical care in the case of chronic ailments and infections.

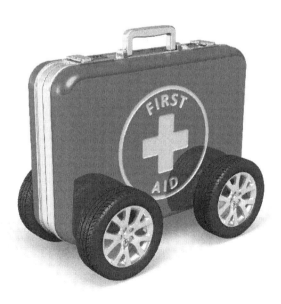

According to research and studies, the consumption of apple cider vinegar is relatively safe for most adults. However as with all natural remedies, there are some cases and instances where the use of apple cider vinegar may lead to some discomfort or complications. It has been noted that the long-term consumption of the averagely suggested one tablespoon (15ml) of apple cider vinegar on a daily basis can lead to low potassium levels within the body; this is despite the potassium content of apple cider vinegar that was mentioned in the previous chapter. According to internet research there has been one report of a case where a person developed very low potassium levels and osteoporosis, which is a chronic disease that results in very weak bones as well as the loss of bone mass; in this particular case the subject had been consuming one cup (250ml) of apple cider vinegar every day for six years.

In another report found while engaging in internet research a subject managed to get an apple cider vinegar tablet lodged in their throat, although this did not lead to any choking or asphyxiation, it was reported that after having this tablet lodged in their throat for thirty minutes, this subject began to experience pain in their voice box and reported to have trouble swallowing for up to six months after the tablet was dislodged.

It was assumed that this was a result of the high acid content of the apple cider vinegar tablet.

In terms of special precautions and warnings when using apple cider vinegar it is important to note that while pregnant and breast feeding is advised that you avoid the use of apple cider vinegar for the treatment and remedy of any ailments as there is not enough information and known side-effects or precautions regarding the use of this remedy during such a time.

When using apple cider vinegar as a means to lower and regulate blood sugar levels it is important to do so with care if you are aware of and are being treated for type two diabetes. Due to apple cider vinegar's ability to lower blood sugar levels there is a possibility that it may lower these levels to a point where they become too low and this can be incredibly dangerous if you already suffer from this chronic illness. It is also very strongly advised that you consult with your physician before beginning the use of apple cider vinegar as a remedy and treatment as it may lead to complications with your existing medical treatments and drugs.

Due to the high acid content of apple cider vinegar it is recommended that one always uses it with care and in moderation when applying it to the treatments of sore throats, teeth whitening and bad breath. There will always be the risk of over-use that can lead to discomfort and a burning of the throat and mouth due to the long-term exposure to the high acidity of the apple cider vinegar.

When using apple cider vinegar as treatment for acne, it is advised to do so with caution as well. The high acid content of the apple cider vinegar can lead to a burning of the skin if used for extended periods of time. There is also the risk of the apple cider vinegar stripping away too much of the skin's naturally occurring oils and sebum resulting in a shock effect whereby the skin will begin producing even more oil and sebum in order to protect itself from the harsh acidity of the apple cider vinegar; this could in turn cause an increase in acne and inflammation.

Once again it would be important to note that it is always a good idea to consult with a medical professional before embarking on and including the use of any home remedy or treatment whether it is in natural or chemical form.

Chapter Three: Apple Cider Vinegar Uses in the Home

In chapter one some of the many uses of apple cider vinegar in terms of healthcare were explored. This chapter aims to show and enlighten you to the many uses of apple cider vinegar in and around the home. You will see how apple cider vinegar is incredibly useful and helpful in everyday household needs and how apple cider vinegar can be used as a cost-effective chemical free home cleaning product.

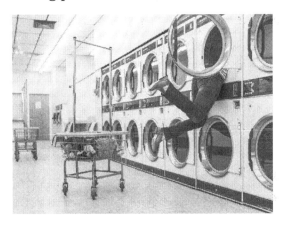

Apple Cider Vinegar to Clean and Sanitize Electronic Equipment:

This particular use applies to both home and office, so it further shows the adaptability of apple cider vinegar. Electronic equipment such as smart phones, telephones, tablets, keyboards, microwave oven buttons, printer buttons, television remote controls; any item that is used on a daily basis and is touched regularly can easily obtain a build-up of bacteria and germs over time. Since apple cider vinegar has a high acid content as well as anti-bacterial properties and due to the fact that it is a natural substance; apple cider vinegar makes a great cleanser and disinfectant for all the above mentioned electronic devices.

To use apple cider vinegar as a disinfectant and cleanser for your everyday electronic devices simply soak a cotton wool pad in neat apple cider vinegar and wipe the device you want to clean with the cotton wool pad, to dry it off use a piece of dry kitchen towel.

Apple Cider Vinegar to Remove Sticky Residue from Household Scissors:

We've all had that moment when we try to use the kitchen or home office scissors and the blades are sticky due to the scissors having been used to cut open packaging that may have had a glue sealant on it or to cut scotch tape. This can be very annoying, but apple cider vinegar is a great remedy to this because of its high acid content it is able to cut through the stickiness of the glue residue that may be on the blades of your scissors.

To use apple cider vinegar to remove glue or stickiness from your house hold scissors soak a cotton wool pad in neat apple cider vinegar and generously wipe the blades of the scissors with the cotton wool pad, making sure to remove any and all glue residue and stickiness.

Apple Cider Vinegar to Remove Candle Wax:

We all love the odd candlelit dinner and there are many occasions when the use of candles can add to the atmosphere and ambiance. There are also those times when we experience power failures and blackouts that lead to the emergency use of candles. Unfortunately due to the nature of a candle and the fact that to use it you are essentially burning and melting the wax that is it is wholly made up of; there are times when this can lead to an unwanted mess and the build-up of candle wax on the surface which you had placed the candle on. If you are using candlesticks or candle holders then there will eventually be a build-up of candle wax on these items as well.

To use apple cider vinegar to remove candle wax, heat the now hardened candle wax with a hair dryer until it has melted to a point where you can remove most of it with a cloth or a rag. There will most likely be stains and residue of candle wax left behind and this is where the apple cider vinegar comes into use. Make up a solution of one cup (250ml) of candle wax and one cup (250ml) of water, soak your cloth in this solution and rub away at the excess candle wax.

Apple Cider Vinegar to Remove Ink Stains:

One of the things that goes hand in hand with having small children around the house is that there will always be times when they disappear out of sight and get up to mischief that can lead to the unintentional defacing of household walls and floors. Almost every parent has had to, at some point, endure finding their walls to have been drawn on with pen or wax crayons and wondering just how to get rid of the stains without having repaint the house.

Apple cider vinegar is a wonderful cost-effective non-chemical way to remove such stains and to do so all you need to do is soak a cloth in neat apple cider vinegar and wipe away at the stains, you will see how they easily loosen and disappear.

Apple Cider Vinegar to Clean and Unclog Household Drains:

The clogging of household drains is something that will always eventually happen and simply cannot be completely avoided. Most of us really become concerned about a clogged-up household drain because we immediately assume that it will require a harsh chemical based product in order to help unclog and clean the drain out.

Apple cider vinegar is a great, cost-effective non-chemical way to clean out and unclog any household drain. Due to its high acid content it is able to cut through grease and detergent build-up within the drain and pipes that leads to the clogging in question. To use apple cider vinegar as means of unclogging your household drains simply mix ½ cup (125ml) of baking soda with one cup (250ml) neat apple cider vinegar and immediately pour down the clogged-up drain. The natural chemical reaction that will occur between the baking soda and the acidity of the apple cider vinegar will result in a kind of fizz-bomb that will release the drain and clean it out.

Apple Cider Vinegar to Remove Mildew from the Bathroom:

The build-up and growth of mildew in the bathroom is unfortunately another one of those household woes that we simply cannot avoid. Due to the constant dampness of a regularly used bathroom we unintentionally create a happy breeding ground for mildew, which can be very frustrating and unsightly.

Apple cider vinegar is a natural and non-chemical option for removing mildew and mildew stains from your bathroom. To remove mildew from your bathroom using apple cider vinegar mix a solution of four cups (1litre) neat apple cider vinegar to four cups (1litre) water in a spray bottle. Generously spray the apple cider vinegar solution over the mildew and allow it to sit for about twelve hours. Wash off with clean water and repeat this process as often as required.

Apple Cider Vinegar to Remove Mildew from your Shower Curtain:

The shower curtain is another happy breeding ground for mildew in the bathroom due to the way in which it tends to form folds when left open; these folds provide damp and dark crevices for the mildew to grow in and a mildew-covered shower curtain can cause many a headache on cleaning day.

To use apple cider vinegar to clean your shower curtain and remove the mildew; take the shower curtain down off the rail and place it in your washing machine. Open the detergent drawer and place ½ cup (125ml) baking soda into the wash cycle compartment and one cup (250ml) of neat apple cider vinegar into the fabric softener compartment of the detergent drawer. Run the washing machine on a full wash cycle. If possible hang the shower curtain out in full sunlight to dry once the washing machine cycle has finished.

Apple Cider Vinegar to Clean Out Your Washing Machine:

A washing machine is one of those household appliances that are used on a daily basis in most households, particularly those with large families. Over time the washing machine can fall victim to a buildup of detergent and fluff from the many loads of washing that it helps you get clean.

Apple cider vinegar is a one of the best ways to clean out your washing machine, because it is a natural substance and non-chemically based any residue of the apple cider vinegar that may remain behind in your washing machine after cleaning will not cause any potential damage or bleaching to the load of laudatory that you do afterward. To use apple cider vinegar as means of cleaning out your washing machine pour two cups (500ml) of neat apple cider vinegar into the drum of the washing machine and run it on a full cycle on the hottest temperature available.

Apple Cider Vinegar to Freshen Up Clothes that Have Been in Storage:

We all know that change of season irritation when we bring our clothes out of storage or the back of the closet only to find that they smell musty and their colors are looking a little dull. This is easily remedied by adding one cup (250ml) of apple cider vinegar to the wash cycle when washing these clothes.

Apple cider vinegar is also useful as a means of preserving and preventing the color of new clothing from running when the garments undergo their first wash. To use apple cider vinegar in this instance, soak the new garment in neat apple cider vinegar for approximately twenty minutes before washing it for the first time. This will help fix the dyes and colors within the fibers of the fabric preventing them from running and fading during future washes.

Apple Cider Vinegar to Help Sanitize Clothes and Very Dirty Garments:

Those of us who lead very active lifestyles and who regularly engage in heavy exercise sessions will know all about the effects of excessive sweating on our workout clothes. Human sweat contains odor causing bacteria and due to its high acidity content it can be rather corrosive to the fibers of that fabrics of your workout gear, and therefore needs to be successfully and completely washed out of clothes after every workout in order to preserve the life and extend the use of these particular garments.

Due to its naturally occurring anti-bacterial properties, apple cider vinegar is a wonderful cost-effective and non-chemical way of ensuring that these particular garments are well sanitized and odor free. To use apple cider vinegar in this instance simply add one cup (250ml) of apple cider vinegar to the detergent drawer when washing these clothes on a long wash cycle in the washing machine. You could also add ½ cup (125ml) of baking soda to the mix in order to ensure that all sweat stains are removed.

This mixture is also very useful as means of removing those stubborn yellow stains that tend to form around the collars and cuffs of shirts. To use the mixture for this purpose mix one cup (250ml) neat apple cider vinegar with ½ cup (125ml) baking soda into a spray bottle, generously spray the solution over the stains and allow it to sit for approximately fifteen minutes before placing the garment into the washing machine for a full wash cycle.

Apple Cider Vinegar to Help Remove wrinkles from Clothes:

If there is one household chore that is guaranteed to be everyone's worst its ironing. We all hate the idea of standing for hour upon hour at the ironing board after washing day, so any other option is always a welcome alternative.

Apple cider vinegar can help remove wrinkles from your clothes without the hardship and chore of ironing. To use apple cider vinegar as means of ironing your clothes, mix one cup (250ml) apple cider vinegar with one cup (250ml) water into a spray bottle. Spritz the wrinkled clothes with the solution and then let them hang to dry.

Apple Cider Vinegar to Clean your Iron:

Unfortunately there are those fabrics that just do better once they have had good iron such as pure cotton. Over time your iron can begin to build up lime scale and dirt from general use. Apple cider vinegar is a non-chemical and cost-effective way to help clean and sanitize your iron in an easy step.

To use apple cider vinegar to clean your iron fill the iron's water reservoir with neat apple cider vinegar and then turn it onto full steam. Allow the iron to sit in the upright position steaming until all the apple cider vinegar has evaporated. Once all the apple cider vinegar has evaporated fill the iron's reservoir with clean water and repeat the steaming process.

Apple Cider Vinegar to Remove Stains from Porcelain Sinks and Bath Tubs:

Over time soap and detergent build-up can lead to stains beginning to appear on the surface and around the porcelain coating of household sinks and bath tubs. These stains can look very unsightly and cause endless frustration on cleaning day.

Harsh chemical detergents such as chlorine based household bleach can cause damage to the porcelain and over time it will cause small cracks to begin appearing in the surface of the porcelain. Although these harsh chemical products are very effective at removing stains from such sinks and bath tubs, they are also harmful to the environment and can cause skin irritations for most people.

Apple cider vinegar is a wonderful alternative to the harsh chemically abrasive detergents and is great for removing such stains. To use apple cider vinegar to remove stains from your porcelain sinks and bath tubs fill the tub or sink with hot water and add two cups (500ml) of neat apple cider vinegar. Allow to soak for approximately twenty minutes before letting the water out and wiping down with a cleaning cloth.

Apple Cider Vinegar to Remove Greasy Residue from your Stove Top and Kitchen Counters:

The buildup of a greasy residue on the stove top and kitchen counters is something that we continually try to avoid, however over time there will still be some sort of buildup due to the steam and general everyday cooking within the kitchen. Chemical based detergents are not always the most desirable option to clean surfaces on which food is prepared and can in many instances cause long term damage to the coating of your stove top and kitchen counters.

Apple cider vinegar is a wonderful non-chemical and non-evasive way of cleaning and removing greasy residue from the entire kitchen. To use apple cider vinegar in this instance mix one cup (250ml) of neat apple cider vinegar with one cup (250ml) of water into a spray bottle. Spray generously over the areas of the kitchen that you would like to de-grease, allow it to sit for approximately twenty minutes before wiping off with a damp cloth.

Apple Cider Vinegar to Remove Water Stains from Wooden Furniture:

As annoying as it is and as much as we try to get our family members and regular visiting guests to use coasters there are always those moments when someone forgets to make sure there is a coaster on the table before they put their drink down. On a hot summer's day this can easily lead to the creation of a water stain that forms as a result of the condensation that builds up on the outside of a glass of cold drink; these water stains can deface your beautiful wooden furniture and cause many a heartache when trying to remove them.

Apple cider vinegar is a wonderful way to help remove such stains without resorting to re-varnishing your wood. To use apple cider vinegar to remove stains such as these from your wooden furniture soak a soft cleaning cloth in neat apple cider vinegar and rub away at the stains. Follow with a good dose of furniture polish.

Apple Cider Vinegar to Clean and Freshen Carpets:

Household carpeting regularly falls victim to the buildup of dirt and odors due to everyday accidents and general household traffic. The odd spill or muddy shoe can also lead to stains and general dirt build up on your carpeting. Due to the fact that household carpeting is made up of fibers it can also easily hold odors. The use of chemical based cleaning products in an attempt to remove these everyday stains can lead to the risk of discoloring your carpets as well as the buildup of a chemical residue that can be harmful to toddlers and crawling infants, as well as pets.

To use apple cider vinegar to clean and freshen your household carpets mix two tablespoons (30ml) of sea salt with one cup (250ml) of neat apple cider vinegar and rub over the area you would like to clean. If the area is reasonably big, double up the basic mixture accordingly. Allow the apple cider vinegar mixture to dry on the carpet and then vacuum as normal.

Apple Cider Vinegar to Clean Stainless Steel Sinks and Cookware:

Harsh water can lead to the buildup of lime scale stains on stainless steel sinks and cookware; this is due to the high lime and chlorine content that is often found within municipal water systems. These stains can be very frustrating and unsightly and very often chemical based detergents can make the problem worse.

Apple cider vinegar is a perfect non-chemical and food safe option when it comes to looking for the right product to help remove such stains. To use apple cider vinegar to remove stains from stainless steel sinks and cookware simply soak a soft cleaning cloth in neat apple cider vinegar and rub it over the stains that you are trying to remove.

Apple Cider Vinegar to Polish Silver:

We all love our silverware and those candlesticks that come out on special occasions, but it can be a serious chore to clean and polish all of these loved household items. Chemical based silverware polish tends to have a very strong odor and can lead to sinus and nasal, as well as skin irritations in most people.

Apple cider vinegar is a great non-chemical and non-irritant option for the cleaning and polishing of your silverware. To use apple cider vinegar to clean and polish your household silverware simply soak a soft cleaning cloth in neat apple cider vinegar and rub over the silverware that you want to clean and polish. If the silverware is really dirty and tarnished you can make a solution of ½ cup (125ml) apple cider vinegar and two tablespoons (30ml) baking soda, soak the silverware in this solution for about two hours and then rinse with clean water before drying off with a dry soft cleaning cloth.

Apple Cider Vinegar to Help Prevent Spots on Your Wineglasses:

There are few things more frustrating than taking out your wineglasses to set the table for a dinner party only to find that they have those annoying spots all over them that come as a result of not being dried properly after having been removed from the dishwasher. This usually results in having to spend more time "polishing" up the wineglasses with a dishcloth before setting them out on the table.

Thankfully apple cider vinegar provides an easy way to help prevent these spots from forming on the glasses in the first place. To use apple cider vinegar to prevent spots on your wineglasses simply add ¼ cup (60ml) of apple cider vinegar to the rinse cycle of your dishwasher.

Apple Cider Vinegar to Remove Stubborn Coffee and Tea Stains from Coffee Mugs and Tea Cups:

Due to the high tannin content of coffee and tea, it has a tendency to stain the porcelain on the inside of coffee and tea mugs. This is a gradual process that happens over time and long term use of the coffee and tea mugs in question. Obviously a chemical based detergent or stain remover is never going to be first choice in this instance due to the fact that they are not necessarily food safe and can cause irritations to many people's digestive systems.

Apple cider vinegar is a natural, non-chemical and very food safe option for removing these stains. To use apple cider vinegar to remove stains from your coffee mugs and tea cups simply mix one cup (250ml) of neat apple cider vinegar with one cup (250ml) of sea salt and fill each coffee mug or tea cup with a batch of this solution. Allow it to soak for about one hour before rinsing out and washing as normal. If you do have a dishwasher it would be helpful to then wash these coffee mugs and tea cups on a very hot cycle.

Apple Cider Vinegar for Cleaning and Disinfecting Cutting and Chopping Boards:

Kitchen cutting and chopping boards make for a very happy and prime breeding ground for bacteria and certain types of fungus. Making sure that your kitchen cutting boards, particularly those that are used to cut meat and fish products, are always sufficiently cleaned and disinfected is an imperative task to continually undertake in your daily kitchen habit. The buildup of bacteria and fungi within the cut grooves that form in your chopping boards with regular use can lead to a number of health problems and very often food poisoning. Any chopping or cutting board that is used to cut raw chicken needs to be thoroughly cleaned and disinfected after every use as there is always the risk of contracting salmonella from raw chicken.

Very often people will soak their chopping and cutting boards in household bleach in order to ensure that they are sufficiently cleaned and decontaminated, however this is a very harsh chemical based detergent that is not necessarily food safe and if the chopping and cutting board is not sufficiently rinsed of all excess household bleach it can also lead to the cause of discomfort and digestive upsets.

Apple cider vinegar is a natural and food safe way of disinfecting and sufficiently cleaning your kitchen chopping and cutting boards. Because of its naturally occurring anti-bacterial and antibiotic properties, apple cider vinegar provides a food safe way of cleaning these everyday kitchen items. To use apple

97

cider vinegar to clean your chopping and cutting boards simply soak them in neat apple cider vinegar for approximately one hour and then run them through the dishwasher on a very hot cycle, alternatively soak them in boiling water for a further hour.

Apple Cider Vinegar to Clean and Deodorize your Refrigerator:

The refrigerator is another of those essential household appliances that can easily fall victim to the buildup of dirt and odors, purely due to its primary use. As much as we all try to avoid forgetting about that tub of leftovers that ends up getting pushed to the back of the fridge and going bad, it's something that happens anyway and can lead to nasty odors staying behind within the refrigerator.

Obviously since the refrigerator is where we store our food, none of us are particularly keen to jump at the chance to clean it out with a harsh chemical-based detergent. Apple cider vinegar, with its naturally occurring anti-bacterial and cleansing properties is a great non-chemical alternative to use to clean and deodorize your refrigerator. To use apple cider vinegar to clean your refrigerator simply mix a solution of equal parts of neat apple cider vinegar to plain warm water; using a cleaning cloth that you have dampened in the apple cider vinegar solution, wipe down the interior shelves and door of your refrigerator before repeating the process on the outside of the refrigerator.

Chapter Four: Apple Cider Vinegar for Beauty and Cosmetic Uses

Apple cider vinegar has many uses when it comes to beauty and cosmetic concerns and since it such a natural and safe to use product it makes a wonderful alternative to the chemical-based and highly fragranced options that the commercial cosmetic industry has to offer to us. It is however important to note that due to apple cider vinegar's high acidity content it can cause irritation and a burning sensations to very sensitive skin. This chapter aims to show and enlighten you to some of the many uses of apple cider vinegar for beauty and cosmetic related concerns.

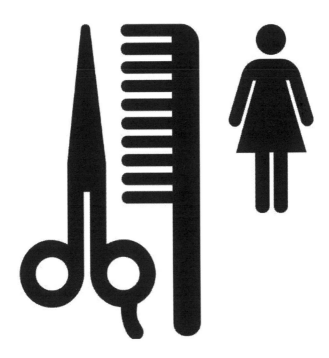

Apple Cider Vinegar for Shiny Hair:

A beautiful shiny and soft main of hair is something that we all long for and always strive to achieve within our beauty regime. Many of the products made available to us by the cosmetic industry are chemical-based and highly fragranced, which can lead to irritations for people with sensitive skin. Also the extended use of styling products can lead to a buildup of these products in our hair causing it to be weighed down and look dull and lifeless.

Apple cider vinegar has a high acetic acid content and is a natural alternative to the products made available by the cosmetic industry for such concern. The use of apple cider vinegar on your hair will naturally remove the buildup of styling products and at the same time strengthen the hair shaft, resulting in a healthy hair follicle that will in turn produce and grow a healthier, shinier strand of hair. Apple cider vinegar will also help to restore the natural pH balance of the scalp and hair shafts resulting in an increase in hair growth and volume. To use apple cider vinegar as a hair tonic dilute ¼ cup (60ml) neat apple cider vinegar into four cups (1litre) of warm water and pour this solution over your hair after shampooing. Leave the solution to sit in your hair for approximately five minutes before rinsing off with cold water, the cold water will seal the hair shaft resulting in shinier hair.

Apple Cider Vinegar as a Facial Mask:

Due to its high acetic acid content as well as its anti-bacterial properties, apple cider vinegar makes a great base for a detoxifying facial mask. The honey that is added to this mixture adds further naturally occurring anti-bacterial properties as well as moisturizing properties for the skin. This natural facial mask mixture also contains bentonite clay which is made up of volcanic ash and is celebrated for its natural detoxifying properties.

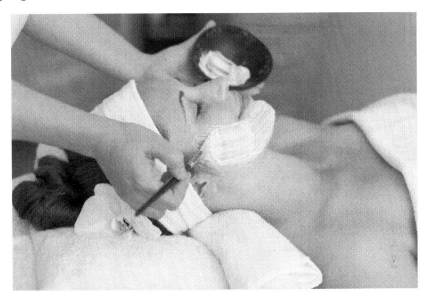

To use apple cider vinegar to make a facial mask mix one cup (250ml) neat apple cider vinegar with one cup (125ml) bentonite clay and one tablespoon (15ml) raw natural honey, make sure you combine all the ingredients into a paste. Apply the mask to cleansed skin and allow it to sit for ten to fifteen minutes before washing off with clean warm water. Pat your face dry and then soak a cotton wool pad in neat apple cider vinegar and wipe the pad over your skin, using the apple cider vinegar as a toner. Follow with your usual moisturizing routine.

Apple Cider Vinegar for a Detoxifying and Moisturizing Bath Soak:

In our fast paced modern lifestyles finding the time to indulge in the activity of soaking in a bath can be very difficult for some of us resulting in the activity becoming more of a treat than a regular part of our routine. However there are so many benefits to soaking our bodies in the warm water of a bath, and when we add a little natural ingredients to help along with the detoxifying and relaxing benefits of such an indulgence, then it makes an even stronger argument for the necessity of including a soak in the bath into our regular beauty routine.

To use apple cider vinegar for a detoxifying and moisturizing bath soak simply two cups (500ml) of neat apple cider vinegar to your warm full bath and soak for approximately twenty minutes.

Chapter Five: Apple Cider Vinegar Recipes

At the end of the day apple cider vinegar is still a food product and therefore this chapter on recipes that use apple cider vinegar even further illustrates how versatile this natural product just is. The recipes in this section will give you a few basic ideas of how to incorporate apple cider vinegar into your daily cooking routines in order to further reap the health benefits and properties that it possesses.

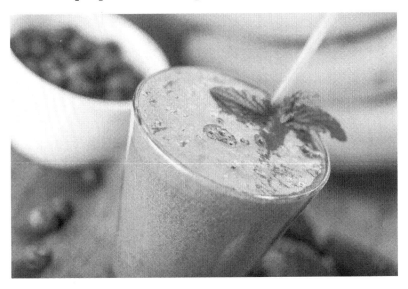

Potassium Punch Smoothie

Bananas are known for their high potassium content and are a very healthy source of easily digestible carbohydrates, making them one the best fruit options for active people and are an amazing pre and post workout food. The dates in this recipe add an extra punch of fiber and vitamin C as well as the essential mineral of iron. The potassium content of the apple cider vinegar adds the extra dose of this muscle restoring and cramp preventing essential mineral. The calcium that is brought to the party by the yogurt makes this smoothie a great source of bone strengthening ingredients as well

Serve One

Ingredients:

- One large banana

- One cup (250ml) Plain fat free yogurt

- ¼ cup (60ml) Dates, roughly chopped

- 1 Tablespoon (15ml) Organic natural peanut butter

- 1 teaspoon (5ml) Organic apple cider vinegar

Instructions:

1. Slice the banana into to the jug of a blender

2. Add the fat free yogurt

3. Add the dates and peanut butter

4. Add the apple cider vinegar

5. Blend until smooth

Apple Cider Vinegar Salad Dressing

Salad dressings don't have to be high in calories and added preservatives; they also don't have to be high in synthetic flavors and chemical additives like mono-sodium-agglutinate (MSG). This recipe will show you how to make a healthy, health benefiting salad dressing using simple and natural ingredients.

Ingredients:

- 1 Cup (250ml) Apple cider vinegar
- ½ Cup (125ml) Extra Virgin Olive Oil
- 1 Teaspoon (5ml) Organic sea salt
- 1 Teaspoon (5ml) Ground Black pepper
- 1 Tablespoon (15ml) Fresh Basil, finely chopped
- 1 Tablespoon (15ml) Fresh or dried Rosemary
- 1 Teaspoon (5ml) Red chili, seeded and finely chopped
- 1 Teaspoon (5ml) Fresh garlic, finely chopped

Instructions:

1. Place all the ingredients into a salad dressing shaker and shake vigorously making sure that you combine all the ingredients together sufficiently.

2. Pour the salad dressing into a glass jar and refrigerate

3. To use: Pour one tablespoon (15ml) of the salad dressing over your favorite salad before serving.

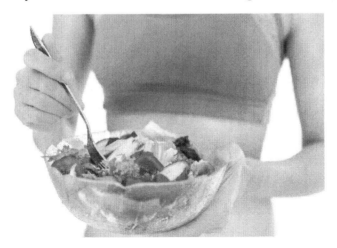

Carrot, Orange and Apple Cider Vinegar Juice

Home made fresh juices are a wonderful way to ensure that you are getting all the health benefits of the fruits and vegetables that you are consuming without any of the added preservatives that are a guaranteed part of commercially packaged juices. Over the last few years we have seen an increase in the popularity of homemade juices and this is a wonderful thing to see as it means that more and more people are taking control of their health and wellness and making sure that they always know what they are consuming. This juice combination is high in antioxidants and vitamin C from the orange juice and the carrot brings along a healthy dose of beta-carotene and vitamin A. The potassium content in the apple cider vinegar, along with its anti-bacterial and antibiotic properties as well as the addition of pure honey make this juice a wonderful idea when fighting off any infection.

Serves One

Ingredients:

- One large orange, peeled and segmented

- One large carrot

- One tablespoon (15ml) Organic apple cider vinegar

- One tablespoon (15ml) Raw organic natural honey

Instructions:

- Using a juicing machine feed the orange segments into the chute

- Feed the carrot into the chute

- Add the apple cider vinegar

- Add the honey

- Juice all together to ensure that all is mixed well

- Pour into a glass and serve.

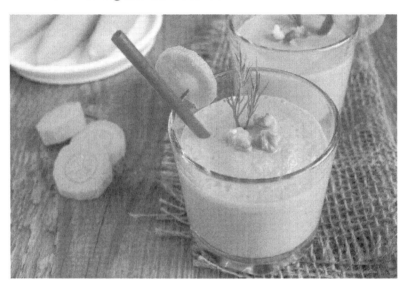

Fresh Ginger Preserved in Apple Cider Vinegar

Fresh ginger has a number of health benefits including anti-bacterial and anti-inflammatory properties. It is also an incredibly useful ingredient in so many dishes from curries to smoothies and desserts. It is always helpful to have some finely chopped ginger close on hand when you are busy preparing your favorite dishes for which ginger is a key ingredient to the overall flavor. In order to preserve the shelf and refrigeration life of pre-chopped ginger we need to add a natural form of preservative. Apple cider vinegar has a high acetic acid content, making it a great natural alternative to any commercial preservative. By adding apple cider vinegar to the jar in which you are keeping your chopped ginger you are naturally extending its shelf life.

Ingredients:

- One cup (250ml) Fresh ginger root, peeled and chunked
- One cup (250ml) Organic apple cider vinegar

Instructions:

1. Place the peeled, chunked fresh ginger root into a food processor fitted with the chopping blade

2. Pulse until the ginger is very finely chopped

3. Place the ginger into a glass jar

4. Pour the organic apple cider vinegar into the glass jar with the ginger, ensuring that all the ginger is covered with the vinegar

5. Keep in the refrigerator and use as needed.

Conclusion

This book shows the many uses and benefits of apple cider vinegar; however since there really are so many it could be argued that this book only touches on these mentioned ways of using and benefiting from this natural product. It is once again necessary to add, in conclusion, that one must always take care when using any product as a natural remedy for health concerns and that it is always a good idea to consult with your healthcare professional before embarking on the use of apple cider vinegar for any health related issue.

PS. One more thing, before you go; could you please **rank this book on Amazon** and let me now your favorite ACV salt tip? It would be really much appreciated and would help me serve you better.

Thanks in advance,

Elena,

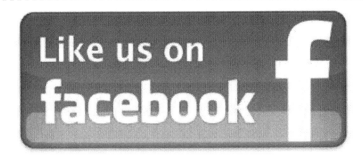

Follow us on Facebook and be the first one to find one about new releases as well as free and discounted eBooks:

www.facebook.com/HolisticWellnessBooks

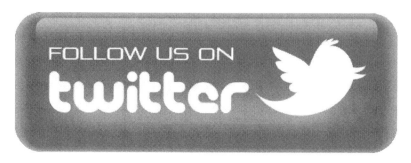

www.twitter.com/wellness_books

Book 3

Ashwagandha

The Miraculous Herb!

Holistic Solutions & Proven Healing Recipes for Health, Beauty, Weight Loss & Hormone Balance

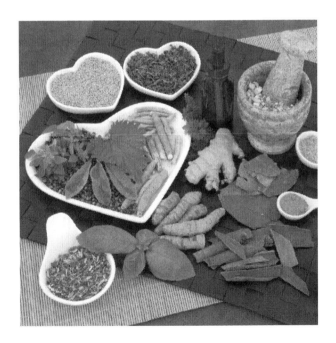

by Elena Garcia

Ashwagandha: Introduction

Ashwagandha is also known as Indian ginseng and is widely used within Ayurvedic healing practices. Ayurveda is an ancient holistic healing practice that originated in the Indian subcontinent. This legendary healing practice began with tales of how the Gods would empower the sages with knowledge around this healing practice that the sages would then pass on to human physicians of the time. As with many ancient healing practices Ayurvedic healing has developed and evolved over the course of the last two millennia into what we know it to be today; however it is still largely based on the ancient traditions and methods.

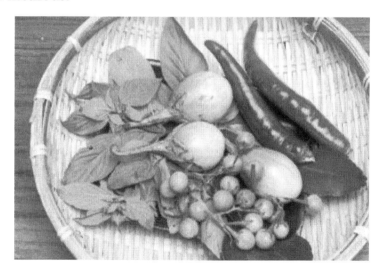

Some Background on Ayurveda:

The theories and practices of Ayurveda are largely based on the use of ancient yet complex herbal compounds, and the evolution of the practice began to introduce the use of mineral compounds within the healing processes as well. The ancient practices of Ayurveda also taught surgical techniques such as rhinoplasty (which is essentially a nose job), basic suturing or the stitching of wounds, and the extraction of foreign objects.

The basis of Ayurvedic practice works on three elemental substances known as *doshas*, these doshas are referred to as *Pitta, Vata and Kapha*, and the belief is that if these doshas are balanced then the body is in a healthy state, but if these doshas are out of balance then the body is in a state of dis-ease and therefore will be needing treatment.

Ayurvedic practice consists of eight accepted components which were derived from ancient Sanskrit literature. These eight components include the practices of the following:

- General medicine and medicine of the body

- The treatment of children (pediatrics)

- Surgical techniques and the extraction of foreign objects

- The treatment of ailments affecting the ears, eyes, nose and mouth (what we know as ENT or ear, nose and throat treatment)

- The pacification of possessing spirits and the extracting of these sprits from those whom they are possessing.

- Toxicology

- Rejuvenation and tonics for increasing lifespan, intellect and strength

- Aphrodisiacs and fertility treatments

When looking at the principles of Ayurveda one will notice that an emphasis is put on the obtaining and maintaining of balance within the body, mind and spirit in order to achieve a holistic state of health and wellness. The practice of Ayurveda cautions people to stay within the limits of reasonable balance and to maintain self-awareness when following nature's urges; therefore one is encouraged to moderate food intake, sleep and sexual intercourse.

Doctors specializing and practicing Ayurveda regard the physical existence, mental existence and personality as unit, with each of these components having the ability to influence each other. This approach is taken when diagnosing and treating a patient's ailments. There is another part of Ayurveda that states that the body has channels which transport fluids and that these channels can be opened up and treated through massage therapy using oils. Unhealthy or blocked channels are thought to cause diseases.

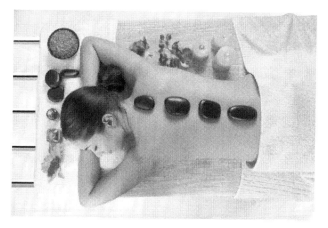

Ayurveda uses eight approaches in order to diagnose illnesses, these approaches include:

- Pulse
- Urine
- Stool
- Tongue

- Speech

- Touch

- Vision

- Appearance

The five senses are always used when approaching diagnosis.

Ayurveda places an emphasis on obtaining and maintaining vitality by building a healthy metabolic system, which consistently possesses a healthy state of digestion and excretion. Ayurveda also places a focus on exercise such as the practice of yoga and meditation. There is also a focus on the maintenance of natural cycles of sleep, waking, working and meditation in order to achieve a state of good health. Personal hygiene, including regular bathing, cleaning of teeth and hair, skin and eye washing are also central to obtaining and maintaining a state of good health.

Ayurvedic treatments include the use of substances that are derived from roots, fruits, seeds, bark and leaves. There are some instances where treatments will call for the use of mineral substances such as sulfur, copper sulfate, lead and gold. Ayurveda will also sometimes use alcoholic beverages as forms of treatment. However many of the most common and well known Ayurvedic treatments are based on the use of herbal remedies.

More about Ashwangandha:

When it comes to the healing practices of Ayurveda, Ashwagandha is considered one the most powerful herbs. The name of the herb comes from the Sanskrit texts and when translated into English means *"the smell of a horse"*, which indicates that it imparts the strength and vigor of a strong stallion. Ashwagandha has been traditionally prescribed to help people recover and strengthen their immune systems after suffering from an illness.

Ashwagandha, although referred to as *"Indian Ginseng"*, due to its rejuvenating properties, it actually has no botanical connection to ginseng at all. Ashwagandha is actually part of the tomato family and is a small, plump shrub that has oval leaves and yellow flowers; the fruit that it bears is about the size of a raisin. This herb is native to growing in the dry regions of India, North Africa, the Middle East and more recently some areas of the United States.

Ashwagandha is known as an adaptogenic herb. Adaptogens are substances such as amino acids, vitamins and herbs that modulate the body's response to stress and/or a changing environment, both of which are consistent aspect of modern day life. Adaptogens are known to help the body cope with and fight against external stressors such as toxins and the environment, as well as internal stressors such as anxiety, insomnia and depression.

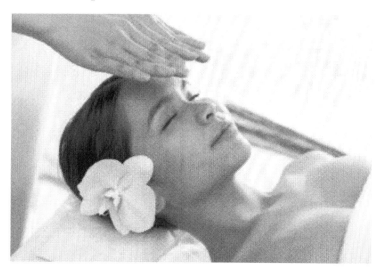

Ashwagandha has many useful medicinal chemical properties such as withanolides, (which are steroidal lactones), alkaloids, choline, fatty acids, amino acids and a variety of naturally occurring sugars. The leaves and the fruit of the Ashwagandha plant possess very valuable therapeutic and healing properties; however it is the root of the plant that is most commonly used in the more Western practices of Ayurveda and its treatments.

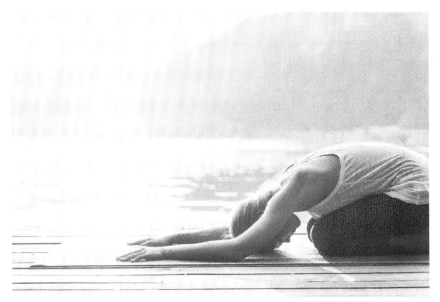

Over the years there have been approximately two hundred documented medical studies based on the Ashwagandha herb and these studies have concluded that some of the healing benefits of this herb include the following key points:

- Protection of the body's immune system; studies have shown that the use of this herb can result in the increase of white blood cell counts

- The treatment and resistance of the effects of stress, both external and internal

- Improvement of cognitive functions such as learning ability, memory and reaction time

- The reduction and treatment of anxiety and depression without the common side-effect of drowsiness that most chemical based treatments come with

- Aids in the reduction of brain cell degeneration

- The stabilization of blood sugar levels and helps to suppress sugar cravings

- The lowering of cholesterol

- Possesses many anti-inflammatory benefits

- Possesses anti-malarial properties

- Boosts and enhances libido and fertility in both men and women

- Useful in the preventative measures taken against cancer

- Helps to fight insomnia

- Helps with the pain management of arthritic joints

- Has a positive effect on the endocrine, cardiac and central nervous systems

- Can help the body maintain healthy thyroid function

- Possesses anti-oxidant properties

Chapter 1:
The Uses and Benefits of Ashwagandha

This chapter will take a more in-depth look at the key points, uses and benefits of the Ashwagandha herb that were mentioned toward the end of the introduction. Each key point will be looked at separately in order to provide as much information regarding the uses and benefits of Ashwagandha with relation to the key point in question. The aim of this chapter is to show how this natural element of healing can be used to fight off, reduce and prevent many of the health risks and conditions that so many people are faced with in today's world.

Ashwagandha for the Immune System:

The modern world has evolved to a time in which we are all living fast-paced lives that involve many unavoidable stressors. These stressors are all around us and are linked to work, home life, school and university, money, health and wellness. Having a healthy immune system allows your body to protect itself from these stressors. Stress, both emotional and physical can put a serious strain on the body and therefore on the immune system, making it important for us to consistently do as much as we can to provide support to this system. As mentioned in the introduction, the practice and principles of Ayurveda include a balance of the mind and spirit together with a balance of the body.

One of the ways in which many of us cope with our daily stressors is through a consistent exercise routine, which is a very good way to combat stress. However for those of us who take our exercise and physical activities to levels that reach further than just everyday moderate exercise, it is important to remember that the fitter you are, the more physical strain your body is capable of undergoing, which will in turn result in your body being under a large amount of physical strain. Physical strain, even the healthy kind that comes in the form of exercise can put the immune system under pressure; therefore it is even more important for very active people and competing athletes to consistently boost their immune systems. Generally if you are choosing to live a healthier lifestyle by keeping active then your overall approach to your health would be one that is holistic and as natural as possible; furthermore, competitive athletes are known to prefer the avoidance of chemical based immune enhancers. This is where Ashwagandha will come in handy as it is a completely natural and safe immune system booster that will ensure that your body can fight off any infections that it may be at risk of contracting due to the physical strain it could be under during times of intense training.

Due to the fact that Ashwagandha has adaptogenic properties it is able to help with the modulation of the body's response to the internal and external stressors that can put the immune system under strain, leading to the risk of contracting everyday viruses and illnesses.

Ashwagandha has the ability to help improve and increase the white blood cell count which is another immune boosting property that it possesses. An optimum white blood cell count is necessary for a strong immune system because white blood cells help to fight infections by attacking viruses, bacteria and germs that invade the body; all things that we are consistently exposed to and cannot avoid as they are all around us in everyday life. The white blood cells could also be referred to as the body's sniffer dogs as they can detect hidden infections and undiagnosed medical conditions. Because the white blood cell count can fall and rise in and out of the healthy range without us knowing, it is important to consistently take measures, through our lifestyles, diets and supplementation to ensure that this particular blood cell count remains within an optimum range. The use of Ashwagandha will be very helpful in this case.

Ashwagandha for the treatment and resistance of the effects of stress, both external and internal as well as for insomnia:

External stressors tend to be the cause of internal stressors. Our daily lives are filled with so many of these stressors that in many cases they are completely unavoidable, but they are controllable.

Examples of external stressors would be our jobs, families, money, school, traffic jams, late busses, broken down trains, leaking pipes, the list could go on forever. Usually many of us can cope with all these external stressors, but sometimes their compound is just far too much to handle and can then begin to cause internal stressors.

Internal stressors are when the body begins reacting to the external stressors and this can lead to many health problems such as cardiac diseases, high blood pressure, diabetes, insomnia, depression and anxiety.

Ashwagandha is very useful in the treatment and prevention of stress and anxiety, helping you to better cope with the external stressors and therefore relieving and preventing the internal stressors that they cause. Ayurvedic healers acknowledge Ashwagandha for its calming effect on the central nervous system, since this herb is also a member of the nightshade family and it is revered within the practice for its ability to help the body adapt to stress and therefore help to prolong life.

Within this ancient healing practice, Ashwagandha has been prescribed over centuries for its ability to ease anxiety, calm panic attacks, alleviate insomnia and reduce depression.

Medical research has revealed that Ashwagandha's relaxant properties are the result of it containing a group of alkaloids known as withanolides. Ashwagandha also contains alkaloids such as sitoindosides and saponins, as well as an assortment of essential minerals, all of which are believed to create a state of relaxation by working on the central nervous system as a depressant, resulting in sensations of relaxation and tranquility; both necessary states in order to achieve consistent and good quality sleepful nights.

Clinical studies in which subject suffering from severe anxiety proved that there was a far more effective decline in, and an increased ability to handle anxiety and stress among those subjects who were treated with Ashwagandha as opposed to those who were treated with psychotherapy alone.

Another clinical study surrounding subjects who were being treated for chronic stress proved that Ashwagandha treatment resulted in a substantial decrease of the stress hormone cortisol.

Ashwagandha for the improvement of cognitive functions such as learning ability, memory and reaction time, as well as the prevention of brain cell degeneration:

Overall sufficient cognitive function enables us to get through daily life far more efficiently then when we are in a constant state of brain fuzz. When our cognitive function is at an optimal level we are able to learn new things faster, remember things more efficiently, and have a much faster and more effective reaction time.

Part of the amazing journey of life is that we are constantly learning new things just by living in the world that surrounds us, however if we are consistently in a state of poor cognitive function we end up just existing rather than living and therefore miss so many of the things that are happening around us on a daily basis; these so-called things hold valuable lessons to our self growth. For example, simply observing the couple sitting next to at the coffee shop can teach you something new about people and their personalities, equipping you with stronger people skills. When you listen to a talk radio show or watch a talk show on television, you are being exposed to new and sometimes very relevant information about the world around you; however if your cognitive function is not firing on all, or most, of its cylinders then you will likely miss out on learning new facts and broadening your general knowledge.

It is well known that sufficient cognitive function is linked to good memory. A good memory is necessary in so many aspects of our daily lives, from remembering to put the food back in the fridge to remembering to lock the front door; a poor memory can lead to accidents and misfortune in so many ways. If your memory function is at an optimal level then you will be able to leave your grocery list at home, but still remember exactly what you need to buy purely because you wrote it down in the first place. Brain cell degeneration will cause you to have low and insufficient cognitive and memory function, which will also affect your learning ability.

In a clinical study surrounding the efficiency of Ashwagandha in promoting and increasing cognitive and memory function, while at the same time naturally reducing the possibility of brain cell degeneration; subjects were given doses of the Ashwagandha herb and then received a bout of psychometric testing. At the end of the two week trial all the subjects showed improvement in their reaction time, visual processing, memory function and overall brain health.

Ashwangadha for the stabilization of blood sugar levels and helping to suppress sugar cravings:

Unstable blood sugar levels and sugar cravings can be the result of many factors, including poor diet and lifestyle, as well as lifestyle related and hereditary diseases such as diabetes.

Studies have shown that the use of Ashwagandha aids in the metabolic process, therefore equipping the body with a stronger digestive system that will be able to efficiently and sufficiently break down all food substances in order to release the energy it is getting from them at a more optimal rate. When our energy levels drop due to hunger and insufficient nutrition, a drop in the levels of healthy sugar within our blood is a result. Blood sugar dips can cause headaches, nausea and in many cases irritability; all of which can lead to sugar cravings.

On the other hand, if our blood sugar rises too quickly, this will send our pancreas into overdrive, causing it to produce too much of the sugar regulating hormone, insulin. Consistent repetition of this state within the body can lead to type 2 diabetes, which is a chronic lifestyle related illness. Ashwagandha is known to help stabilize blood sugar levels keeping them from rising or dipping too fast or too high.

When our digestive systems and metabolisms are functioning at their peak then our bodies are able to reap all the nutritional benefits of the food that we are consuming. However it is important to note that even though Ashwagandha has been proven to aid and increase the metabolic and digestive process, it cannot erase the side-effects of a poor diet since a poor diet is a poor diet whichever way one looks at it. Ashwagandha would therefore be used as a supplement and a treatment in order to help get these systems within the body back on track and functioning at their peak.

Ashwagandha for the lowering of cholesterol, blood pressure and reduction of cardiac diseases:

Cholesterol is known as the silent killer as many of us don't know whether or not we are suffering from higher than normal or dangerous levels of bad cholesterol. High cholesterol can be caused by a number of factors that include hereditary disorders, bad lifestyle and dietary choices and chronic stress.

Ashwagandha has been known to effectively treat high cholesterol due to its ability to aid in the metabolic and digestive functions, helping the body to efficiently break down all the food that we eat. However, as with type 2 diabetes, if your high cholesterol is a result of a poor diet, Ashwagandha can only be used as a supplementation, preventative and treatment for your high cholesterol, and you would have to take all the factors that cause this state into consideration in order to effectively manage it.

Chronic stress can lead to high cholesterol due to the fact that it causes an increase in the stress hormone cortisol. Cortisol is known to affect a number of things within the body, including the healthy levels of cholesterol, therefore even if you are living a healthy life and following a nutritionally sound diet you could be at risk of high cholesterol if you are under chronic and server amounts of stress. This is where Ashwagandha's ability to help relieve stress has a double sided effect; by using this herb as a means to combat and manage your chronic stress situation, you are also in turn using it to help lower your cholesterol levels.

A combination of chronic stress and high cholesterol, as well as high blood pressure can lead to cardiac diseases by putting immense strain on the heart muscle and its regular function.

Again there are a number of factors that can lead to high blood pressure and cardiac diseases, many of which include poor lifestyle and dietary choices as well. These too are conditions that can be managed without the use of chemical based drugs; through a lifestyle change that focuses on achieving sound health through diet, exercise, and stress management one can easily keep all these conditions under control. Ashwagandha can help in this situation on a number of levels due its stress relieving ability, as well as its digestive enhancing properties.

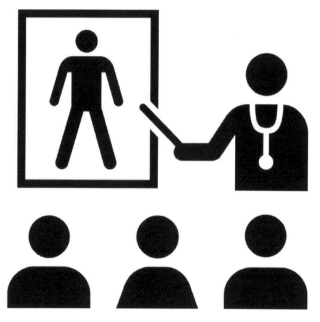

When one looks at high blood pressure on its own; there are many cases in our modern times where it is a result of our stressful lifestyles, here again it can be managed and prevented by the calming effects that come with the use of Ashwagandha.

Ashwagandha as an anti-inflammatory and for the pain management of arthritic joints and gout:

Inflammation within the body and its cellular makeup can lead to a number of health problems that include chronic cardiac diseases and a compromised immune system. Ashwagandha is known widely for its anti-inflammatory properties and therefore is a great addition to your daily routine in order to boost overall health and wellness in this aspect.

For those who suffer from arthritis and painful joints, Ashwagandha is a great remedy due to its anti-inflammatory properties. Arthritis is synonymous with an acid build up and inflammation within the joints and is usually caused by factors such as it being hereditary, a long-term side-effect of an injury, and the normal unavoidable aging process.

Gout is similar to arthritis in that is also caused by a high acidity within the joins and the body in general. This high acidity level can lead to pain and inflammation, which can be very effectively managed and remedied with the use of Ashwagandha.

Ashwagandha to boost and enhances libido and fertility in both men and women:

Ashwagandha is known for its potency when treating low libido and boosting the function of the fertility system in both men and women. When we have a healthy sex drive, we have a healthy reproductive system.

Fertility and the ability to conceive is very much affected by our stressful lives; there have been many cases where couples have been unable to conceive despite trying for a long time, and then suddenly once they relax about the situation the woman in the relationship is pregnant. Chronic stress can have a huge influence on fertility, and that's where Ashwagandha's stress reducing and stress treating properties play a role in the boosting of fertility. Also, when we are highly stressed and exhausted the last thing on our mind is intimacy, therefore our sex drive will naturally take a plunge.

Ashwagandha not only helps fertility and libido through its stress relieving properties, but also through its ability to promote healthy blood flow, therefore resulting in the treatment of impotence in men and the lack of lubrication in women. When our blood flow is pumping optimally around our system then our genitalia and reproductive systems are provided with enough healthy oxygen-rich blood, resulting in an increase in libido and fertility.

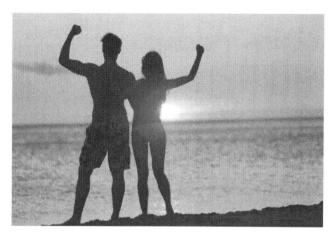

Ashwagandha for the prevention of cancer and as an anti-oxidant:

Due to its well-known high anti-oxidant properties and the fact that it is a known adaptogen, Ashwagandha has been shown, through numerous studies, to possess cancer fighting and cancer preventing properties.

Many of the cancer cases we hear about today are a result of the highly stressed lives we lead. Chronic stress leads to a compromised immune system and in so many cases it can, and does, lead to depression. There is an age old belief that unhappiness can lead to cancer, as the mind and soul is so strongly linked to the body.

Studies have shown that Ashwagandha's ability to increase the immune system's artillery which is our white blood cell count; it can be incredibly beneficial when used in conjunction with, and as part of, cancer treatment. These studies have also shown that Ashwagandha has the ability to promote the effects and efficiency of chemotherapy, resulting in a faster recovery time of certain types of cancers.

Further studies have shown that due to the alkaloids that make up the biochemical structure of Ashwagandha, it has the ability to reduce and prevent the growth of cancer tumors. It has also been discovered that this herb possesses cytotoxic properties against lung, colon, central nervous system and breast cancer lines.

Ashwagandha for the treatment of thyroid function and hormone rebalancing:

Due to its adaptogenic properties, Ashwagandha has been linked to, and in many cases proven to, aid in the optimum functioning of the thyroid and adrenal system, therefore rebalancing the body's hormonal system as well.

Ashwagandha has been known to help people with both hypo and hyper thyroid problems as it has been proven to treat and help both an over-active and an underactive thyroid gland. Ashwagandha was found to further benefit thyroid function due to its ability to greatly reduce lipid peroxidation through its ability to promote the destruction of free radicals that cause cell damage.

Due to its ability to fight and treat chronic stress, Ashwagandha has been found to be very supportive and useful in treating and strengthening the adrenal system, which is the system that is responsible for releasing the hormones cortisol and adrenaline; both of which are related to stressful situations. When you are under a chronic amount of physical, emotional and psychological stress your adrenal glands can take strain causing a condition that is known as adrenal fatigue. Adrenal fatigue can have a negative effect on the other hormones in your body such as progesterone which can then affect your fertility and cause you to age faster.

Ashwagandha's stress relieving, sedative, and carminative properties help to treat this adrenal fatigue and therefore promoting the rebalancing of your body's hormonal system, leading to more energy, increased libido and fertility, a stronger immune system, lowered and regulated blood sugar, lowered and regulated blood pressure, lowered and regulated cholesterol, and overall sound health for body, mind and spirit.

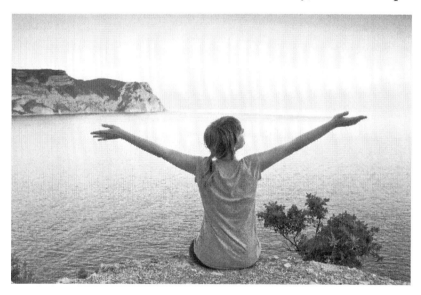

Chapter 2:
Side-Effects and Precautions of using Ashwagandha

As with anything in this world, be it good or bad for the system, there are always going to be exceptions when it comes to the tolerance of certain medications, foods, and drinks. Although Ashwagandha possesses so many useful benefits to our overall health and the treatment of life's everyday upsets, there are also some side-effects that may occur while using this miracle herb, as well as some precautions that need to be taken into account. This chapter will look at these side-effects and precautions in order to make sure you are fully equipped with all the necessary knowledge around the use and application of Ashwagandha at all times.

Firstly it is good to note that the long term safety and side-effects of using Ashwagandha as an oral treatment are not completely known, however it is known that use of the herb as an oral medicinal compound in the short term has proven to be safe in general circumstances, but there is the possibility that overdose of the herb can lead to stomach upset, diarrhea and vomiting in some cases.

However it is advised to take certain precautions under the following circumstances:

- **When Pregnant or Breastfeeding:**

Due to the fact that there is not enough known about the use and side-effects of using Ashwagandha while breastfeeding, it is advised that it is completely avoided during this time. It is also suspected that there is a possibility that the use of

Ashwagandha during pregnancy may lead to miscarriages so it is best to avoid the use of the herb completely during pregnancy.

- **In the case of Diabetes:**

Although Ashwagandha has many healing and useful properties when it comes to the prevention and treatment of diabetes, there are also cases when it has been known to interfere with prescribed Western medications for this particular lifestyle ailment. This interference has led to causing the blood sugar levels to drop too low, which can be very dangerous. It is always advised to consult with your physician before commencing treatment with Ashwagandha in order to ensure that you will not be putting yourself at any risk of the herb causing an interference with your existing treatment.

- **In the case of high or low blood pressure:**

Due to Ashwagandha's ability to help lower blood pressure, there is the risk that it may reduce blood pressure to a level that is too low in people who are already suffering from lower than normal blood pressure. Therefore you should take serious precautions when using Ashwagandha if you know that you have low blood pressure or if you are taking any medication for blood pressure in general. Again it is <u>highly advised that you consult with your physician</u> before commencing treatment with Ashwagandha to make sure that you are not putting yourself under any unnecessary risks.

- **In the case of stomach ulcers:**

There is a strong possibility that the use of Ashwagandha can cause irritation to the gastrointestinal tract. If you suffer from any kind of gastric disorders such as irritable bowels syndrome, crone's disease or a stomach ulcer it is advised that you either avoid the use of Ashwagandha completely or consult with your physician before commencing any treatment that involves the use of this herb.

- **In the case of Auto-Immune Diseases:**

If you suffer from or have been previously diagnosed with any of the auto-immune diseases such as multiple sclerosis, lupus, rheumatoid arthritis or any other disorder that is known to attack the immune system it is advised that you avoid the use of Ashwagandha as there is the strong possibility that it may increase the symptoms of these diseases. **Once again it is best to consult with your physician** if you are considering including Ashwangandha into your daily routine in order to reap its other benefits. There is an exception to every rule.

- **Ashwagandha and Surgery**

Ashwagandha has the ability to calm the central nervous system, which is a very good thing when using it as a treatment for stress and trauma, however in the event of surgery and post-surgery recovery there is the possibility that it may cause the central nervous system to slow down too much. There is also a strong concern that Ashwagandha may interfere with or cause a reaction with the anesthesia and other medications that are administered before, during and after surgical procedures. It is advised that you stop taking Ashwagandha at least two weeks before any scheduled surgical procedure **and of course you should consult with your physician**.

- **In the event of Thyroid Disorders:**

Even though Ashwagandha has many benefits when treating thyroid and hormonal imbalances and disorders, there is still the risk that it may increase thyroid hormone levels to a level that is not optimal. If you are using Ashwagandha as a treatment for thyroid or hormonal disorders it is advised that use it cautiously and **always consult with your physician** before commencing treatment. If you are taking thyroid or hormonal medications then it is advised that you avoid the use of Ashwagandha all together.

Chapter 3: Mouth-Watering Smoothie Recipes using Ashwagandha

The best, most efficient and easiest way to use and incorporate Ashwagandha into your daily life is by adding it in its powdered form to your smoothies. Ashwagandha powder is available at most health stores, pharmacies, and online. This chapter focuses on smoothie recipes that combine all the nutritional benefits of fruit, seeds, nuts, coconut; and in some cases super foods such as raw cocoa powder, Maca powder and Spirulina powder. All the recipes are completely vegan friendly so they are suitable for all walks of life.

As mentioned in the introduction; Ashwagandha is an herb that is used widely within the Ayurvedic practices of healing and balance of mind, body and soul, one of the key aspects of Ayurveda is sound nutrition and well balanced diet, these smoothies will help you achieve that. Many of the ingredients included in these recipes will not only help boost your immune system with their high nutritional content, but their high fibre content will also help you to achieve a healthy, well-working digestive system. Further benefits of the ingredients that have been included in these recipes include libido and fertility boosting properties.

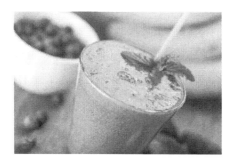

Libido Boosting Café Mocha Kick-Start Smoothie

Studies have shown that coffee reduces the odds of erectile dysfunction in men by increasing blood flow to the genitals, and its caffeine content will give you an energy boost. Raw Cocoa has been proven to contain the highest amount of anti-oxidants within one food source, and is a well-known natural anti-depressant. Maca is an ancient super food known to fight fatigue, increase energy, endurance and strength. Maca also stimulates the pituitary gland, which is responsible for secreting sex hormones. When combined with Raw Cocoa, Macca has synergistic effect. Cinnamon is used in Ayervedic healing because of its ability to promote healthy menstruation, and nourish the female reproductive system. Bananas are high in potassium and are known as a great natural energy source. The addition of Ashwagandha to this smoothie rounds off all the health benefits, making it not only good for boosting your libido and sex drive, but also adding a holistic approach to the ingredients.

Serves One:

Ingredients:

1 Cup (250ml) Almond milk

½ Cup (125ml) Organic filter coffee, preferably chilled

1 teaspoon (5ml) Tahini

¼ teaspoon (1.25ml) Vanilla Essence or extract

¼ teaspoon (1.25ml) Ground Cinnamon

1 teaspoon (5ml) Raw Cocoa Powder

1 teaspoon (5ml) Maca Powder

1 teaspoon (5ml) Ashwagandha Powder

1 medium sized banana

1 Tablespoon (15ml) chopped raw Hazelnuts

Instructions:

- Pour the almond milk and coffee into the jug of your blender.

- Add the Raw Cocoa, Ashwagandha and Maca Powders.

- Add the ground cinnamon, chopped Hazel nuts and Tahini.

- Add the vanilla essence or extract.

- Slice the banana into the jug.

- Blend until smooth.

- Since the almond milk does not require refrigeration, you can either drink this smoothie immediately, or pour it into a shaker to take away.

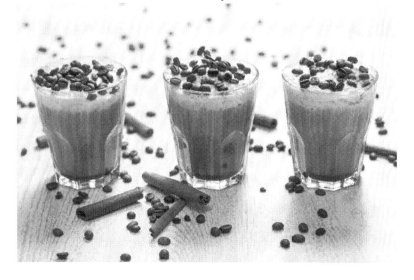

Apple, Date and Chia Smoothie

According to the healing principles of Ayervedic diets, apples are believed to work wonders for the sex drive, while dates help by combating fatigue, both fruits are high in the anti-oxidant vitamin C, so they add a cancer-fighting punch to the mix. Chia seeds are an ancient Mayan super food prized for their ability to provide sustainable energy. Chia seeds are also high in omega 3 fats, which are essential to a healthy female reproductive system and a strong immune system. Oat milk is high in calcium, which is essential for strong bone structure.

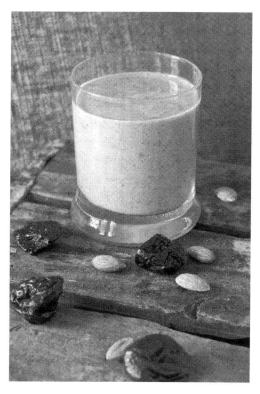

This smoothie uses a combination of oat and Chia seed milk, and requires a little preparation of ingredients prior to putting the actual smoothie together.

Serves One:

To make the Chia Seed Milk:

Ingredients:

- 2 Tablespoons (30ml) Chia Seeds

- 1 Tablespoon (25ml) Chopped raw almonds

- ½ teaspoon (2,5ml) vanilla essence

- ½ teaspoon (2,5ml) ground cinnamon

- 2 ½ Cups (750ml) water

Instructions:

- Mix the Chia Seeds, almonds and ground cinnamon together in a large jug.

- Add the water and vanilla essence.

- Set aside until the Chia Seeds have expanded to make a liquid with a milky consistency.

To make the smoothie:

Ingredients:

- 1 Cup (250ml) Oat Milk

- 1 Cup (250ml) Chia Seed Milk

- 1 Medium sized apple, cored and diced (peeling the apple is

- Up to you)

- 1 teaspoon (5ml) Ground Cinnamon

- 1 teaspoon (5ml) Ashwagandha powder

- 1 teaspoon (5ml) Tahini

- ¼ Cup (60ml) Chopped Dates

Instructions:

- Pour the oat and Chia Seed milks into the jug of your blender.

- Add the diced apple, chopped dates, Tahini, Ashwagandha powder and ground cinnamon

- Blend together until smooth.

- This smoothie will be best consumed immediately.

Coco-Pine Alkaline Ayurvedic Smoothie

Pineapple is a great source of vitamins C, B1 and B6; it is also high in manganese and folic acid, which is a good booster to the functioning of the reproductive and immune system. Coconut milk and desiccated coconut provide essential fats, as does the Tahini paste, these essential fats are known to help increase good cholesterol levels and lower the bad ones, and therefore they are incredibly useful and healthy to the cardiac system and functioning.

Serves One:

Ingredients:

- 1 Cup (250ml) Coconut Milk

- 1 Cup (250ml) Diced pineapple

- 1 Tablespoon (15ml) Desiccated coconut

- 1 Teaspoon (5ml) Tahini

- 1 Teaspoon (5ml) Freshly ground ginger root

- 1 Teaspoon (5ml) Ashwangandha powder

Instructions:

- Place the coconut milk and diced pineapple into the jug of a blender

- Add the desiccated coconut, Tahini, and ground ginger

- Add the Ashwangandha powder

- Blend until smooth

Chocolate Apple and Banana Secret Smoothie

This smoothie packs the energy boosting benefits of apple, which is a fruit known for its high pectin content making it a lower GI option and a great choice when looking to sustain your energy throughout the day. Apples are also high in anti-oxidants and essential minerals. Bananas are high in potassium and are also a great source of slow releasing energy and dietary fibre, adding to the energy boosting and sustaining properties and benefits of this recipe. The Raw cocoa not only adds a chocolaty taste, but also brings along all its powerful antioxidants, known as a super food, raw cocoa is believed to be the only food source to contain such a high level of anti-oxidants in one serving.

Serves One

Ingredients:

- One small banana
- One small apple, cored and diced (peeling is optional)
- 1 Cup (250ml) Almond milk
- 1 teaspoon (5ml) Ground Cinnamon
- 1 teaspoon (5ml) Maca Powder
- 1 teaspoon (5ml) Raw Cocoa Powder
- 1 teaspoon (5ml) Ashwagandha powder
- ¼ teaspoon (1.25ml) Vanilla essence
- 1 teaspoon (5ml) Natural almond butter

Instructions:

- Slice the banana into the jug of a blender.

- Add the diced apple

- Add the almond milk

- Add the Maca powder, Raw Cocoa and Ashwagandha powders

- Add the almond butter, ground cinnamon and vanilla

- Blend until smooth.

Minty Mango Anti Cancer Spirulina Smoothie

Among other nutrients, mangos give a good dose of vitamin E, which has been known to help improve sexual health. Spirulina is a super food made from a natural alga, and is very high in proteins, anti-oxidants, essential amino acids, omega 3s and is also very rich in vitamins and minerals. There is a lot of research that shows coconut milk to beneficial in the prevention of a number of cancers, particularly prostate and breast cancers as it is very alkaline forming in the body.

Serves One

Ingredients:

- 1 Cup (250ml) Coconut Milk

- 1 Cup (250ml) Diced Mango

- 1 Tablespoon (15ml) Chopped fresh mint leaves

- 1 teaspoon (5ml) Spirulina Powder

- 1 teaspoon (5ml) Ashwagandha powder

Instructions:

- Pour the Coconut Milk into the jug of a blender.

- Add the diced mango and fresh mint leaves

- Add the Spirulina and Ashwagandha powders

- Blend until smooth

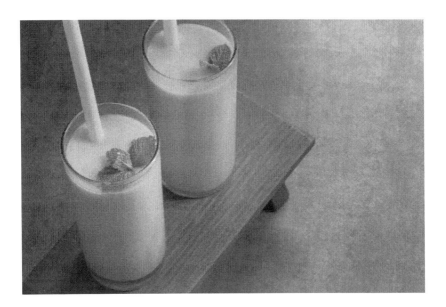

Strawberry Banana Oat Milk Smoothie

Strawberries are rich in folate, which is a B vitamin recommended for optimum pre-natal health, they are also high in anti-oxidants and offer many other nutritional benefits such as immune boosting qualities and a high vitamin C content. With the addition of the Shilajit powder, which is another herb that is used within Ayurvedic practices for the treatment of fertility and low libido, this smoothie is great for both men and women who are trying to conceive, especially considering that it also included all the fertility boosting benefits of the Ashwagandha powder. The energy provided by the banana will give you that extra boost and great dose of potassium.

Serves One

Ingredients:

- 1 Cup (250ml) Oat Milk
- 1 Cup (250ml) Chopped Strawberries
- 1 Medium Sized banana
- 1 teaspoon (5ml) Shilajit Powder
- 1 teaspoon (5ml) Ashwangandha Powder
- 1 Tablespoon (15ml) Chopped Raw Almonds

Instructions:

- Pour the Oat milk into the jug of a blender
- Add the chopped strawberries and slice the banana in to the jug as well
- Add the chopped almonds, Ashwangandha and Shilajit Powders
- Blend until smooth

Rice Pudding Smoothie

Rice milk is a great source of B vitamins and antioxidants. Blueberries also pack a good dose of vitamins, minerals and antioxidants and cancer fighting properties.

Serves one:

Ingredients:

- 1 Cup (250ml) Rice Milk

- 1 Cup (250ml) Blueberries

- 1 teaspoon (5ml) Ground Cinnamon

- 1 teaspoon (5ml) Ground Baking spice mix

- 1 teaspoon (5ml) Ashwangandha Powder

- 1 teaspoon (5ml) vanilla essence or extract

- 1 Tablespoon (15ml) Tahini

Instructions:

- Pour the rice milk into the jug of a blender

- Add the blueberries

- Add the ground cinnamon, spice mix, Ashwagandha Powder and vanilla. Add the Tahini and blend until smooth.

Super Antioxidant Anti Age Pomegranate Berry Smoothie

Goji Berries are not only super high in antioxidants, and cancer fighting properties. Acai berries originate from Brazil and are believed to increase overall energy and sex drive. Pomegranates are more widely known for their anti-aging properties, but have also been known to help improve skin health and are renowned for their ability to reduce the effects of aging within the cellular makeup of the body. Brazil nuts are thought to be one of the most concentrated sources of selenium, which has been linked to the improvement of testosterone levels as well as cognitive function. This recipe also contains Chia Seed milk, which will have to be made in advance.

Serves One:

To make the Chia Seed Milk:

Ingredients:
- 2 Tablespoons (30ml) Chia Seeds
- 1 Tablespoon (25ml) Chopped raw almonds
- ½ teaspoon (2,5ml) vanilla essences
- ½ teaspoon (2,5ml) ground cinnamon
- 2 ½ Cups (750ml) water

Instructions:
- Mix the Chia Seeds, almonds and ground cinnamon together in a large jug.
- Add the water and vanilla essence.

To Make the Smoothie:

<u>Ingredients:</u>

- 1 Cup (250ml) Chia Seed Milk
- 1 Cup (250ml) Almond Milk
- ¼ Cup (60ml) Goji Berries
- ¼ Cup (60ml) Acai Berries
- ¼ Cup (60ml) Pomegranate berries
- 1 medium sized banana
- 1 Tablespoon Chopped Raw Brazil Nuts
- 1 teaspoon (5ml) Maca powder
- 1 teaspoon (5ml) Ashwagandha Powder
- 1 teaspoon (5ml) Raw Cocoa Powder
- 1 teaspoon (5ml) Ground Cinnamon
- 1 teaspoon (5ml) vanilla essence

<u>Instructions:</u>

- Pour the Chia Seed milk, almond milk and vanilla essence into the jug of a blender.
- Add the all the berries and pomegranate
- Slice the banana into the jug
- Add the chopped Brazil nuts, cinnamon, Maca, Cocoa, and Ashwagandha powders
- Blend until smooth.

Coco-Pine and Cashew Nut Smoothie

Cashew nuts are high in heart healthy fats and protein. Pineapple is known for its high anti-oxidant and vitamin C levels. The coconut milk and cream bring along some extra heart healthy fats to the party as well as a tropical taste.

Serves One

Ingredients:

- 1 Cup (250ml) Coconut Milk

- ½ Cup (125ml) Coconut Cream

- 1 teaspoon (5ml) Vanilla essence or extract

- 1 Cup (250ml) Diced Pineapple

- 1 Tablespoon (15ml) Desiccated Coconut

- 2 Tablespoons (30ml) Chopped Raw Cashew nuts

- 1 teaspoon (5ml) Ground Cinnamon

- 1 teaspoon (5ml) Maca Powder

- 1 teaspoon (5ml) Ashwangandha Powder

Instructions:

- Pour the vanilla, coconut milk, and coconut cream into the jug of a blender

- Add the diced pineapple

- Add the desiccated coconut, raw Cashew nuts, ground cinnamon, Maca powder and Ashwangandha powders

- Blend until smooth

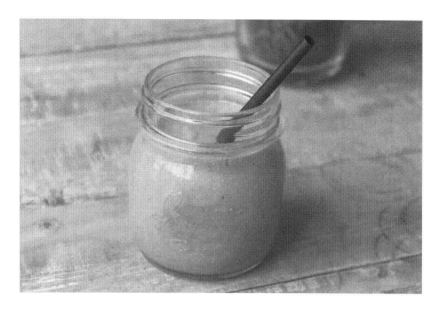

Green Apple and Pistachio Smoothie

This recipe uses green apples in particular purely for the colour aspect, don't be tempted to peel the apple for this one, as the rind will add extra fibre and colour to the end result. Certain studies have shown, that along with their cholesterol lowering abilities, pistachio nuts are also a great source of protein. Oat milk not only adds a creamy texture to this recipe, but it is also high in calcium and B vitamins.

Serves One:

Ingredients:

- 1 Cup (250ml) Oat Milk
- 1 large green apple cored and grated.
- 1 medium sized banana
- 2 Tablespoons (30ml) Chopped raw pistachio nuts
- 1 teaspoon (5ml) Spirulina powder
- 1 teaspoon (5ml) Ashwagandha Powder
- 1 teaspoon (5ml) Vanilla Essence

Instructions:

- Pour the Oat milk into the jug of a blender
- Add the grated apple and slice in the banana
- Add the chopped pistachios
- Add the Spirulina and Ashwagandha powders
- Add the vanilla
- Blend until smooth.

Carrot Cake Smoothie

The high fibre content of this smoothie will give you sustained energy. The carrots add a dose of vitamin A, and the Pecan nuts a high protein and zinc content which helps to balance hormones, by adding the Ashwagandha powder to this recipe this smoothie is a great option when you want to achieve an optimum hormonal balance within your body.

Serves One

Ingredients:

- 1 Cup (250ml) Rice Milk
- ½ Cup (125ml) Coconut Cream
- ½ Cup (125ml) grated carrot
- ½ Cup (125ml) chopped pineapple
- 2 Tablespoons (30ml) chopped raw Pecan nuts
- 1 teaspoon (5ml) ground cinnamon
- 1 teaspoon (5ml) baking spice mix
- 1 teaspoon (5ml) vanilla essence
- 1 Tablespoon (15ml) Raw oats
- 1 teaspoon (5ml) desiccated coconut
- 1 teaspoon (5ml) Ashwagandha powder

Instructions:

- Pour the rice milk, coconut cream and vanilla essence into the jug of a blender.
- Add the grated carrot and chopped pineapple

- Add the chopped pecan nuts, ground cinnamon and spices
- Add the desiccated coconut and raw oats
- Add the Ashwagandha powder and blend until smooth

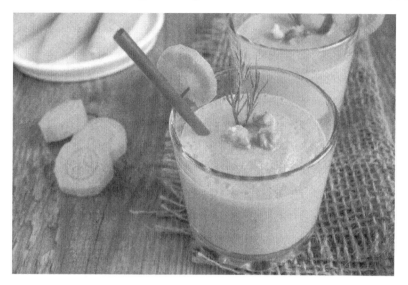

Peach Almond and Banana Smoothie

Almonds are high in omega 3 fats and contain the amino acid l-arginine, which helps transmit neurotransmitters to the brain, increasing sensations and cognitive function. Peaches are high in vitamin C, which is believed to boost libido in women, and their blood circulation boosting properties will help increase arousal. The addition of the Ashwagandha powder to this smoothie mix makes it a great source of libido boosting ingredients for any woman who is trying to increase her sex drive and conceive.

Serves one

Ingredients:

- 1 Cup (250ml) Almond Milk

- 1 Large fresh peach, pitted and diced

- 1 medium sized banana

- 2 Tablespoons (30ml) chopped raw almonds

- 1 teaspoon (5ml) vanilla essence

- 1 teaspoon (5ml) Maca powder

- 1 teaspoon (5ml) Ashwagandha powder

- 1 teaspoon (5ml) Raw cocoa powder

Instructions:

- Pour the almond milk into the jug of a blender

- Add the diced peach and slice the banana in

- Add the chopped almonds, Maca, Ashwagandha and Cocoa powders

- Add the vanilla

- Blend until smooth.

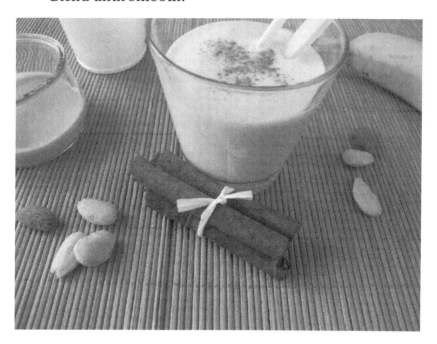

Potassium Punch Aztec Aphrodisiac Smoothie

Avocados were used by the Aztecs as sexual stimulants. This is a fruit that is high in folic acid and its healthy fat, potassium and vitamin B6 content boost hormone production as well as the strength of the immune system. Together with the nutritional benefits of the bananas, this smoothie combination is sure to give you long lasting energy. The high fibre content along with the lubricating benefits of the heart-healthy fats found in the avocado make this creamy smoothie a great stimulant for a healthy, well-working digestive system as well.

Serves One

Ingredients:

- 1 Cup (250ml) Rice Milk

- ½ Cup (125ml) Diced avocado

- 1 medium sized banana

- 1 Tablespoon (15ml) Tahini

- 1 teaspoon (5ml) Maca Powder

- 1 teaspoon (5ml) Ashwangandha Powder

Instructions:

- Pour the rice milk into the jug of a blender

- Add the diced avocado, and slice in the banana

- Add the Tahini, Maca and Ashwangandha powders

- Blend until smooth

In Conclusion

This book shows that there are many, many health and wellness benefits to the super herb known as Ashwagandha, furthermore the benefits of the Ayervedic practice and its healing methods are shown to be an efficient and natural way to achieve a holistic state of health for the mind, body and soul.

As mentioned in chapter 2, regarding the side-effects and precautions that need to be taken around commencing treatments that include the use of Ashwagandha, it is always advisable to consult with your physician before doing so as it is never a good idea to put your body and health at any risk.

We hope you enjoyed this book and are excited about taking care of your mind and body in a holistic way!

If you have a second, please rank this book on Amazon and post a short comment. Your opinion is very important to us and we would love to know your favorite recipe so that we can create more similar resources for you to enjoy.

Remember to take care of your lifestyle. Simply focus on one little change at a time and be good on yourself. Try to spend more time in nature. Disconnect from computers and technology as much as you can. Consider joining local yoga classes and embrace a positive mindset. Try to give yourself the luxury of sleep. We know that it may sound boring to many people- but going to bed earlier is one of the best natural cures you can imagine and it's free.

If you suffer from insomnia, the good news is that with Ashwagandha you can fight it very effectively without utilizing chemical medications and pills. For better results, we recommend you start using essential oils that are proven to help you relax: lavender, verbena, chamomile, sweet orange are great for that. Simply add 3-4 drops of your chosen essential oil to 1 tablespoon of coconut oil and add this mix to your bath, or use it for a self-massage after showering/bathing.

Book 4

Ayurveda

Ayurvedic Essential Oils & Aromatherapy for Amazing Relaxation, Beautiful Skin and Tremendous Healing

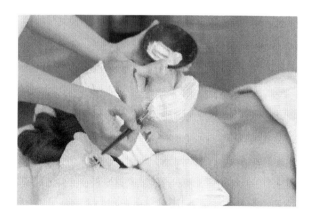

By James Adler and Elena Garcia

Disclaimer:

A physician has not written the information in this book. Although Ayurvedic therapies are generally safe to use, if you suffer from any serious medical condition, are pregnant, or on medication you should consult your doctor (preferably a doctor who specializes in oriental medicine) first to see if you can apply it. It is also advisable that you visit a qualified Ayurvedic Doctor so that you can obtain a highly personalized treatment for your case, especially if you want to make Ayurveda a part of your lifestyle. This book is for informational and educational purposes only.

All information in this book has been carefully researched and checked for factual accuracy. However, the author and publishers make no warranty, expressed or implied, that the information contained herein is appropriate for every individual, situation or purpose, and assume no responsibility for errors or omission. The reader assumes the risk and full responsibility for all actions, and the author will not be held liable for any loss or damage, whether consequential, incidental, and special or otherwise that may result from the information presented in this publication.

If you are pregnant or have any serious health condition, do not use any aromatherapy treatments described in this book without consulting with your physician and aromatherapy practitioner first.

"Self massage with aromatherapy ignites your internal pharmacy, and stimulates all the systems of your body" Deepak Chopra

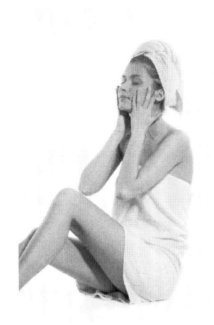

Introduction to Aromatherapy and the Ayurvedic Lifestyle

Thanks for purchasing our book. We are Elena and James, a married couple interested in holistic health and oriental therapies. A few years ago we decided to immerse ourselves in the amazing world of Ayurveda (the traditional natural medicine that originated in India about 5000 years ago). We first went on a month long vacation to India and traveled the country. We got really interested in the food, the culture, and their methods of healing. James had done his basic introductory training in Ayurveda before (he is a health coach and a life coach), but for me, Elena, it was like a new discovery. We like our Western aromatherapy, but Ayurveda makes it much more holistic.

We have decided to put this booklet together to share our passion for Ayurvedic Wellness with you and to show how easy it is to incorporate some highly therapeutic healing rituals into your everyday life. We especially recommend this book for beginners in both aromatherapy and Ayurveda, but we also hope that if you are not new to those topics, you will also find some new tips, motivation and inspiration.

We stand by the belief that one thing is to know and another is to apply. This is the mistake that we have both done, for example, we knew so many great wellness tips from Ayurveda but we did not take any action to commit ourselves to it. Hence, sometimes the excess of knowledge does not equal to putting theory into practice. This is why we would like to encourage you to use this book to actually do your own Ayurvedic healing spa, meditate, relax and heal yourself and those around you on a regular basis.

Finally, we would like to add that we are not Ayurvedic doctors or gurus. We are here to spread the word of Ayurveda in a practical way. We believe that life is all about learning. Actually, the more we learn, the less we think we know! We are students of Ayurveda and will always be. This is a never ending story.

One of our Ayurveda teachers from Kerala used to say, "All those Westerners come here to learn some practical Ayurvedic solutions. They want to learn more about their own bodies and minds. They also want to know how to undo the damage that very often they have done to themselves by their fast-paced Western lifestyle. They tell me that I know a lot. To be honest, I always tell them that I know very little. I am still learning from my master and I always tell him that he does know a lot. He, in turn replies that he does not know that much and it's his master who knows a lot and he looks up to...and so on and so forth..."

We hope that you understand what we mean by the learning process. This is what Ayurveda is all about; it is the science of life, getting to know yourself and even those around you. There are also emotions involved as well as your mental attitude; it's not only about the physical health. It's all interconnected.

As you probably already know, or heard, *Ayurveda* is essentially an ancient system of Hindu traditional medicine native to India. It originated as an extension of the *Rigveda*, contrary to some beliefs where it is seen as a part of *Atharva-Veda*. *Charaksamhita* and *Susrutha Samhita* are the oldest and foundational Ayurvedic texts.

Ayurveda approaches the enumeration of our body in 5 typical elements, also known as the P*anchabhuta*. These 5 elements are:

- Fire (Agni)
- Air (Vayu)
- Water (Jal)
- Ether (Akasha)
- Earth (Prithvi)

Ayurveda also has 7 classic tissues, also known as D*hatu*, which are:

- Plasma or *rasa*,
- Blood or *rakta*,
- Muscles or *masa*,
- Fat or *meda*, bone or *asthi*,
- Semen or shukra and
- Marrow or majja

This system of medicine follows the principle of maintaining a balance in the three humors, or doshas, as they are called.

This balance means a state of health, in contrast to imbalance, which is suggestive of a disease or a disorder. Notice that our modern, Western medicine does not include this concept, as it assumes that you are perfectly healthy if there are not any symptoms visible and that you are ill when the diseases manifests itself. Then, of course, our Western doctors prescribe something that is supposed to kill the symptoms, but very often causes havoc and imbalances to the rest of the organs.

The oriental medicine is more about being persistent in observing one's body and making it one's goals to take good care of oneself. Ayurveda works with plenty of natural therapies ranging from balanced nutrition and herbs to aromatherapy and massage. There is also yoga and meditation.

Each natural therapy can be adopted in a different way according to your dosha type.

Let's have a look at Ayurvedic Doshas, this step of getting to know ayurveda is like getting to know yourself, your body, mind and emotions. This is a process where you just have to ask yourself dozens of questions, and you should also pay attention and observe your own body, something that we oftentimes neglect (Western standards of life are so awful!).

Various imbalances can arise out of lack or excess of either of the following humors or *Doshas*:

- **Vata**- This belongs to the idea of the 'impulse principle' or the nervous system.
- **Pitta-** This belongs to the transforming principle and primarily works according to the secretion of the bilious humor, which is crucial in direct digestion and metabolism. This humor essentially deals with the digestive system of the human body.
- **Kapha-** This is the body fluid principle which deals with mucous and its function in lubrication and nourishment.

Doshas are not like a visible concept that can be touched and easily categorized. We all consist of them, and one of them is our prevalent dosha. We are born with some kinds of predisposition, for example James is vata/pitta type and Elena is kapha type. In order to achieve balance, and therefore the ultimate wellness, one should know their prevalent dosha and learn how to use ayurvedic natural therapies and tailor them to their own needs. If you are a beginner, we know that it all may sound really complicated, but as they say: "different strokes for different folks" Makes total sense, right?

So, let's dive into the doshas, it's fun as you can try to figure out which one would be your prevalent dosha. Of course, to be 100% sure, you would need to book an appointment with an Ayurvedic doctor or practitioner so that they can diagnose you after asking you dozens of questions and doing some tests (again, it's fun, we really encourage you to play the doshas game!).

Vata- Vata people are thin, very often tall as well, and energetic. They have creative minds that ponder easily and they love new experiences like travelling and meeting new people. They are always on the go and doing something but they may also experience a sudden drop of energy. They oftentimes have cold feet and hands.

When unbalanced, they may experience constipation, headache, anxiety and insomnia. They don't benefit from irregular lifestyle patterns and they need to stick to their healthy routine like balanced meals, regular work shifts and sleep patterns. Vatas can get angry very easily. But they also know how to forgive and don't hold a grudge.

On the physical level, vata people normally have dry skin and dry, fragile hair.

Once the vata dosha is out of balance, the following conditions may manifest: lack of appetite, arthritis, weakness, and digestive problems.

Pitta- Pitta people are excellent leaders, they love being in charge. They are also very intellectual and are excellent decision makers (Vatas, on the other hand, are really creative but very often in two minds when it comes to making a decision).

Pittas can be short-tempered and always have to be right. They have strong digestion and so very often they think they can neglect their nutrition and eat whatever they want.

They are great speakers and know how to express themselves, they can often be too direct and so offend some people.

On the physical level, pitta people are usually of medium size /weight. They very often have ginger or red hair and fair complexion. They may be also prone to balding.

Unlike vatas, they always have warm hands and feet, this is why it is recommended they use cooling oils for self-massage.

Kapha- Kapha people have big bones and strong body. They have an excellent stamina but are characterized by such features as being slow, solid, steady and soft. They tend to be really calm and organized as well as supportive and helpful for other people. They like leading a peaceful and organized lifestyle and are not fond of changes, in fact it's hard for them to end a relationship or quit a job.

They also have tendency to accumulate old things at home (they love staying at home!) and are also prone to excess weight, water retention, depression, and very often stubbornness. They find it very difficult to take action so as to embark on something new.

They love to sleep excessively and to take naps.

An increase or decrease in any of these doshas shall lead to an imbalance. This imbalance is rectified by finding a *srota,* or the source of this alteration. This alteration is explained by Ayurveda as the lack of healthy channels for the smooth functioning of these humors. Aromatherapy massage oils, or *Swedana* (steam therapy) are just an examples of natural ayurvedic therapies used to bring balance.

Buddhism and Hinduism play a major role and have a major influence on the central principles of Ayurveda. An emphasis is given to balance whereas suppression of urges is unhealthy and can lead to sickness.

Here is a really funny example: when you suppress a sneeze, it can lead to shoulder pain. However, it also advocates that certain urges should be maintained in a reasonable manner, like moderate intake of food, adequate sleep and sexual intercourse.

Excess can be harmful, and so can be the lack of something. Westerners, when stressed out or confused, very often resort to alcohol, drugs and sex, but usually end up more stressed out and missing the balance. Ayurveda can help you learn more about you and prescribe a myriad of natural therapies that will make up the lack of certain dosha, but at the same time will reduce the possible excess of another dosha.

Practices derived from *Ayurveda* are a part of the Complementary and Alternative Medicine (CAM). This form of medicine is either complementary or alternative since it delineates itself from the conventional, scientific form of medicine. Along with Ayurveda, *Siddha* medicine and traditional Chinese medicine also form a part of Complementary and Alternative Medicine.

Aromatherapy, as a holistic therapy, takes into account the physical and the mental well-being, along with lifestyle and eating habits. Coined by Frenchman Gaffoseer in 1936, this practice uses essential oils extracted from plants for the healing and therapeutic purposes. Aromatherapy may be considered a relatively new therapy in our Western culture, perhaps even a little bit over-hyped these days, but it has been used for ages and it forms an integral part of Ayurveda

This treatment involves addressing the imbalance in a patient, especially with respect to cognitive function, mood or mental health. This form of treatment is found to be useful in the treatment of various common complaints related to the respiratory system, the lymphatic system, circulation, skin, hair, and the nervous system.

In fact, aromatherapy has the capacity to slow down the sympathetic system, which is the system responsible for the fight or flight reaction and, at the same time, it stimulates the parasympathetic system, which is the one responsible for pleasant feelings and emotions. Hence, aromatherapy can have almost an immediate positive effect on your general well-being.

According to Dr. Light Miller, of Ayurveda and Aromatherapy fame, a disease has 6 stages, which are defined as:

a) Accumulation
b) Aggravation
c) Dissemination
d) Relocation
e) Manifestation
f) Disruption

She asserts that imbalance can occur at the Accumulation stage due to improper lifestyle and eating habits. This is in contrast to the western idea of medicine, where the imbalance is acknowledged at the Manifestation stage.

Aromatherapy Massage

This branch of Aromatherapy is known as **_Abhangaya,_** which is a daily massage routine; it has also been practiced by Indian women for their infants for many years.

In India, new born babies are massaged with oils until the age of three, as it enhances circulation of blood, mobility of joints and builds their immune system. This has often been seen as a practice of the social rural culture.

I am sure you have heard of Indian head massage. If you ever go to India, make sure you treat yourself to it on a daily basis and experience how good it feels. So much better and real energy stimulating than our Western cup of coffee!

Of course, you don't have to go to India to try Indian head Massage; there are plenty of highly qualified practitioners in the Western countries, and thanks to this book, you will learn enough about Ayurvedic Aromatherapy to perform one at home whenever you need it!

The most famous Indian Head Massage guru is Narenda Mehta.

Narendra Mehta was born blind and developed an amazing sense of touch.He left his native India to study physical therapy in London. During his studies he was surprised that the Western physical therapy massage overlooked the importance of head massage and personalized aromatherapy (physiotherapists do not usually work with oils). He decided to get back to his roots and take pride in his ethnicity. He managed to combine what he was taught in India (Indian Head Massage is like a tradition that is passed on from generation to generation) with his knowledge of anatomy and physiotherapy.

Narendra Mehta is the author of the book *The Power of Touch*, and he and his wife are teachers dedicated to Indian Head and Face Massage. If you are ever in London, you can visit their Champissage Centre (Champi, or Champissage, is another name for Indian Head Massage).

- *"Incorporate Aromatherapy in your everyday living as a holistic treatment to promote overall well-being and healing on the physical, emotional and spiritual levels." - Deepak Chopra*

Chapter 1: Understanding the Origins of Aromatherapy

The first evidence of the use of aromatherapy is believed to be the burning of tree gums, leaves, needles, and fragrant woods in ancient times. The beginning of this practice can be linked to the discovery that some woods used for making fire (such as cedar and cypress) filled the air with their scent when they burned.

It may sound surprising to you, but Aromatherapy, the term itself, was coined in the late 1920's, but in reality, for about hundreds and even thousands of years, roots of aromatic plants were used for making perfumes, incense and other medicinal purposes. Rather aromatic plants were used for medicinal and healing purposes way back in time as opposed to aromatic oils.

Some people may object when they hear that aromatherapy has been used for thousands of years. This is because they only associate aromatherapy with the essential oils that are labeled and ready to use, something that our Western, scientific world is used to.

We usually tell them to trace some history; many ancient cultures were using aromatherapy daily for all kinds of rituals, they would also start developing their own aromatherapy and naturopathy for different ailments.

The Egyptians have been credited with the invention of the first distillation equipment around 3000 BC. It involved the infusion of rudimentary oils with herbs, the product of which was used in rituals, cosmetics, medicine, and perfumery. It was years later that Hippocrates (widely regarded as the "Father of Medicine") first studied how different essential oils had an effect in healing and for medicinal reasons, and hence promoted the use of these oils.

In India, the use of aromatic herbs can be traced through history, and was called *itr,* meaning 'fragrance' in Arabic. The history of *itr* is as old as the Indian civilization itself. The earliest instance of distillation of *itr* has been found in the Ayurvedic text called *Charaksamhita*. In 7th century AD, the *Harshacharita* mentions the use of fragrant agar wood oil.

Coming to the modern era, the field of aromatherapy was established as a field of science in an accidental discovery by Rene Maurice Gatttefosse, a French chemist, who, as we have already mentioned, is responsible for coining the term 'Aromatherapy'.

What happened is that Gatttefosse suffered from a burn injury while working in the lab. As a reflex, he dunked his hand in a tub of lavender oil, which was the nearest liquid. The burn healed quickly and without any scarring. This led him to research essential oils extensively. In 1937, Gatttefosse published the book titled *Aromathérapie: Les Huiles Essentielles Hormones Vegetales.*

This may be a little bit off topic now, but yesterday we had a family picnic in the local woods. We got back with several mosquito bites each. We applied one drop of lavender essential oil on each bite and both the swelling and the redness disappeared overnight. We are almost healed now! We also use bergamot oil as a mosquito repellent and on mosquito bites to stimulate healing. More on different modes of application in the following chapters!

While the original work was in French, later an English translation titled as *Aromatherapy* was published; this is in print even today.

Other famous Western Aroma Therapists are: Dr. Jean Valnetm who relied on Aromatherapy for treating WWII Soldiers, Madame Marguerite Maury, a biochemist from Austria who used aromatherapy in cosmetics and eventually for massage purposes, and Robert B Tisserand, who wrote the first book on Aromatherapy in English.

Though Aromatherapy is widely used across the world for healing and curing certain illnesses, in ancient times essential oils were used for mystical experiences. For example, frankincense has always been used for mystical meditation.

"Frankincense has, among its physical properties, the ability to slow down and deepen the breath...which is very conductive to prayer and meditation" (from Davis, P. London School of Aromatherapy notes)

Rosemary was used by Romans in religious or wedding ceremonies, in food and in cosmetics, and the Egyptians used it as incense. Since the study in Aromatherapy, Rosemary is now used for stimulating hair growth, boosting mental activity, reducing pain and relieving respiratory problems. As you can see, one essential oil is really multifunctional and can be used for treating a range of conditions.

In the same manner, thyme leaves that we find abundantly in the kitchen and our kitchen gardens is widely used in Aromatherapy. Thyme oil has been found useful in the treatment of digestive and respiratory conditions. So yes, there are many plant materials and herbs, which you use for cooking and other purposes that are vastly used in Aromatherapy.

The following chapters will help you discover some really refreshing, holistic self-care tips...

Chapter 2: Ayurvedic Aromatherapy as a Holistic Medicine

Unlike modern medicines, Ayurvedic Aromatherapy believes that a healthy body is the result of a perfect communion between the physical and spiritual self. It takes into consideration your everyday lifestyle and teaches you how to change your habits. The most extraordinarily striking part is that it gives your illness a chance to heal.

The underlying methodology behind all Ayurvedic treatments is a firm belief in the fact that <u>prevention is better than cure</u>. To a large extent that stands absolutely true in the case of most ailments. The focus therefore, is to prevent the germination of a disease rather than fretting later. Aromatherapy, therefore, can be seen as essential when people are struggling with stress issues and physical challenges almost on a daily basis.

Ayurvedic Aromatherapy uses essential oils to set into motion its larger objective of healing and recuperation, and it also ensures a healthy balance between a proper diet, exercise, herbs, meditation and yoga (of course, the focus on this book is on aromatherapy only). All this in turn leads to the treatment of a number of diseases and prevention of yet more in number.

Like we said earlier, Aromatherapy is an example of a perfect coupling of medication and nature. It goes back to nature and uses natural ingredients for treatment of various problems and deformities. Now, wouldn't you like to opt for natural treatments as opposed to modern day medicine to get relief from your illnesses?

It indeed is a growing challenge to the monopoly of the conventional medicines used over time as people are becoming more and more aware of Ayurveda and its therapeutic qualities and going the natural way. This is the reason that an entire tourism industry is booming in countries like India, Egypt and China, which specializes in natural oriental medicine. It's quite funny for us now, but one of our teachers used to say:

"I do not understand how come so many Westerners who are wealthy (from the authors: even if you think you are not rich, you will be considered rich when you go to countries like India) and come from developed countries know less about proper self-care than my 7 year old son! How come they allowed so much negligence to take place and now they really need to get back to the roots!

I have also have students from Europe, North America and Australia who actually decided to stay in India and quit their jobs and break away from their Western social status. They were blown away by the quality of life that is achieved both thanks to how much money you are making, but also because WHO YOU BECOME and HOW YOU TAKE CARE OF YOURSELF AND THOSE AROUND YOU".

The commonly used ingredients in Ayurvedic Aromatherapy include herbs and oils extracted from numerous plants that have medicinal value. The oils extracted are supplied to the body in different ways, including adding them in bathing water, inhaling them, or using them in diluted form (essential oil diluted in good quality carrier cold-pressed oil).

If you are new to aromatherapy, and Ayurveda, let's have a look at some aromatherapy definitions that we will be using throughout this booklet:

Essential Oils (EO): these can be described as pure essences extracted from different parts of fruits, trees, flowers and stems.

Even though they are called "oils", they are not oily at all.

Before employing essential oils topically, via massage, it is of paramount importance to first dilute them in good quality vegetable base oil (these are oily).

Test on a small area of skin first to make sure you are not allergic, because some people will break out in rashes/blister if it turns out they are allergic/sensitive to certain extracts. And that really takes the fun out of the whole experience.

The general rule of a thumb, that is typical of the English school of aromatherapy and one that we recommend to beginners, is to use up to 5 drops of your chosen essential oil, or oils, in one tablespoon of carrier oil (vegetable oil).

Ok, we understand that a tablespoon may differ on size sometimes, so let us tell you that by saying one tablespoon we mean about 15 ml.

Vegetable Oils (VO): These are the carrying oils. You will need them as a natural base for your massage treatments. They will be able to penetrate your skin and let the essential oils do their job.

Don't use poor quality mineral oils. Work only with natural vegetable oils.

Some Popular Ayurvedic Essential Oils (our favorites!):

- Lavender
- Bergamot
- Betel Leaf
- Black Cumin
- Black Pepper
- Birch
- Bakul Attar

- Rosewood
- Sambrani

Popular Ayurvedic Vegetable Oils:

1. Sesame oil
2. Jojoba oil
3. Coconut oil
4. Grape seed oil

Ayurvedic Aromatherapy does wonders in treating ailments as effectively as it fights stress and anxiety. This is the reason why more and more stressed out Westerners are turning towards it. It is a common practice these days to use Aromatherapy in close conjunction with massage therapy, phytotherapy and the likes.

The best part of Aromatherapy is that the treatment offered is personalized, because each person has a unique constitution, so in a way you will get a personalized Aromatherapy treatment based on your physical traits and needs.

Warm and energizing oils are used for people who are at a higher risk of headaches, hypersensitivity and insomnia. Sharp scents are avoided and warm scents are combined with calming oils. An amalgamation of oils extracted from camphor, cinnamon along with soothing ones like jasmine, rose and sandalwood are considered apt. This particular category of people falls under the *Vata* type (James).

The *Pitta* type of people who are prone to acidity, skin problems, inflammation, ulcers and fevers are easily agitated. They are treated by exposing them to cooling and soothing fragrances like sandalwood, rose and mint. For proper treatment, the carrier suited is coconut oil as opposed to sesame oil which is used as a carrier in case of the *Vata* people. The *Kapha* types who are predisposed to respiratory problems are said to benefit from light and warm oils like basil and cedar used with extremely light carrier oils. Sharp stimulating fragrances are also effective.

Ayurvedic Aromatherapy has made a tremendous contribution to the field of preventative care. It caters to a number of problems including acne, cold and flu, skin allergies, heart diseases and Alzheimer's disease. Herbs and essential oils provide prevention by building a stronger immune system. If you are harrowed by constant headaches or colds, then you should definitely opt for Aromatherapy treatments as a first line of defense.

It would not be wrong to categorize the technique as a holistic one that cares for everything. In fact, it is a great source of mental strength and goes a long way in providing a soothing effect on your mind.

There are a lot of stress-relieving oils that are used in Aromatherapy. These include:

- lavender,
- bergamot
- clary sage

Aromatherapy goes a long way in detoxifying the body, which is extremely important. Using Aromatherapy oils for bathing, massaging and rubbing the neck and abdomen has the potential for relieving the body of unnecessary toxins.

"By oil massage the human body becomes strong and smooth-skinned; it gains resistance to exhaustion and exertion"

Charak Samhita

AROMATHERAPY PRECAUTIONS

Aromatherapy General Precautions

Aromatherapy is a very safe and easy therapy to use, but keep in mind that there are certain precautions:

- Remember to wash your hands after applying aromatherapy massage;

- Do not apply the essential oils in their pure form as they may cause an allergic reaction. Instead, use blends that contain 2-5% essential oils diluted in good-quality cold-pressed oil;

-After using citrus oils, like for example lemon, verbena, bergamot, orange etc. avoid direct sun exposure, even up t0 8 hours after the treatment

- Do not apply oils after surgery (unless you have consulted with a doctor) or on open wounds or rashes of unknown origin;

- Do not use the oils after chemotherapy (unless suggested by a doctor);

- Keep the oils away from the eyes and mucus membranes;

- Use the oils only topically (unless you have consulted with an aromatherapist who specializes in phytoaromatherapy);

- Avoid rosemary, thyme, Spanish and common sage, fennel and hyssop if you suffer from high blood pressure;

- Do not apply the treatments described in this book on babies or infants. It doesn't mean that aromatherapy can never be used on babies and infants, but extremely low concentrations should be used. Always consult with a medical or naturopathy doctor first;

- After an aromatherapy massage always remember to wash your hands;

- Make sure that you research the brand, read safety instructions for each individual oil you buy/use and check the expiration date;

- Store your blends in dark glass bottles, preferably in a cool, dry and dark place and remember to use within a maximum of one month after mixing.

Chapter 3: Mechanism and Mode of Application

Using aromatherapy is a real pleasure to the senses, it can offer an immediate relief for stressed out bodies and minds!

Vaporized odor molecules released by essential oils float in the air and then reach the nostrils, and quickly dissolve in the mucus, which is on the roof of each nostril.

The process may seem a little bit technical, but in reality it is pretty simple. The olfactory epithelium situated underneath the mucus paves way for the molecules to reach the olfactory receptors that are special receptors and the neurons detect the odor. The odor formed there is transferred to the olfactory bulbs situated at the back of the nose.

The olfactory bulbs are of primary importance. This is so because they are home to the sensory receptors, which actually form a pivotal part in the brain. The message catalyzed by the essential oils aim to cure the patient of a particular disease. It then gets transmitted to the brain center, and these in turn have a substantial impact on emotions, memories and other higher levels of the consciousness.

In simple terms, the scent of certain oils and herbs has a soothing, calming effect and can cure certain illnesses. These herbs. when used in the right manner, can help build immunity and also help fight against many illnesses.

The mechanics behind Aromatherapy are still not completely understood and requires a lot more work to uncover its full potential. However, one thing you can be sure of, the aromas induced by the essential oils have an influence on the brain and an impact on the **limbic structure** (it is responsible for pleasant feelings and emotions) this can help you in keeping many conditions at bay, without the help of any synthetic drugs or medication.

There is also more to it- imagine that you get back home from work after a really stressful day. You treat yourself to a nice aromatherapy bath and then you massage your body with your chosen vegetable oil with a few drops of your chosen Ayurvedic essential oil, or oils. What will happen is that the oils will penetrate your skin and will finally get absorbed to your circulatory system. They will then continue their healing job of detoxifying and stimulating your immune system.

Of course, during the aromatherapy massage (both self-massage and one you can get from the hands of an experienced Ayurvedic masseuse), you will also experience the pleasure of aromas, as we have previously discussed. So, to sum up, it's like 2 in 1 treatment. The effect on your olfactory tract and the limbic system of the brain is almost immediate while when applied on the skin, it may take a few hours to penetrate your system and do the healing. This is why, after aromatherapy massage, we recommend you do not shower for about 8 hours. We are both in habit of doing our personalized aromatherapy massages before we go to sleep.

We don't use any body lotions or milks (unless they are organic), we only use natural oils that we know work for us. We don't like lots of different products accumulating on our bathroom shelves, we prefer just a couple of cold pressed vegetable oils that we use as a base for our treatments and a range of essential oils that we mix and blend with the vegetable oils to personalize our treatments.

The reason is simple- we don't want any artificial ingredients on our body. You may be wondering: "does it mean I can't use any creams or lotions"?

The answer is- you can use them as long as they are pure and organic.

Natural lotions and creams are great as a base for aromatherapy treatments.

We normally use vegetable oils or aloe vera gel though. We just got used to using them on a regular basis and we find them multifunctional.

Different Modes of Application

Ayurvedic Aromatherapy is quite diverse in its application and therefore can be made available through a number of means, depending upon your needs, time, work and requirements. The three widely accepted modes of application are topical application (we have already mentioned massage and self-massage Abhyanga treatments), direct inhalation and aerial diffusion.

1. Aerial diffusion is similar to environmental fragrance. Its purpose is to fill a room with a natural fragrance. You could make use of certain simple methods and devices to carry out the diffusion effectively. Simple tissue diffusion is easy, convenient and easily transferable.

It is very instrumental in a workplace or a public place as you could easily complete it by putting drops of aroma on a tissue and the aroma itself diffuses as you move around.

Steam diffusion however, is a faster means of diffusing an aroma in a room. The steam helps to heat the oil and thereby bring about a faster diffusion of oils in the air. Candle diffusion also works for a lot of people, and hence you see a lot of variety of aromatherapy candles in stores and wellness clinics. However, the essential oils are generally flammable, so this method demands a lot of caution (essential oils need to be kept away from the direct flame). The aroma is not long-lasting and sometimes, due to the heat, its effect might fade away faster. Yes, but if you are just looking for relaxing your senses, then candles may do the trick.

There are many commercial products available these days that can help in diffusion. These include lamp ring diffusers made of terracotta or brass. The best part about them is they are not expensive; rather they are efficient to carry out a desired purpose. Fan diffusers are also available in the market, and they help to diffuse the aroma in the air. Electric heat diffusers are effective in spreading the fragrance in a larger area and are also more productive when it comes to thicker oils. Oil nebulizers can also be considered as one of the many options available in the market. This is an excellent way to create a nice atmosphere in your house and improve your well-being in only a few seconds.

2. Direct inhalation is a means of disinfecting the respiratory system. It helps decrease congestion, increases and enables expectoration and also psychologically enhances your moods and energies. Among the many advantages of direct inhalation are stimulation of the brain and immune system, mood enhancement and relaxation.

In this method, you breathe the evaporating oil straight in. It could be done easily by placing a few drops of your chosen essential oil on the wrists and rubbing them together. The hands should then be cupped over the face carefully protecting the eyes and thereafter the oil should be inhaled three to five times.

One could also inhale directly from the bottle- just open it and take a few deep aroma breaths. I, Elena, always carry bergamot essential oil in my bag as it helps me relax and think clearly. I am very often exposed to stress because of work and my business. Aromatherapy is soothing for me and imparts a calming effect on my body, mind and emotions. I never let the tension accumulate; I prevent it from taking over my body. I know that thanks to aromatherapy self-care that I do on a regular basis, I am more successful and productive at work, with my clients and enjoying time with my family.

James finds relief in oils like clove or basil. We both think that they have mysterious, masculine scent.

Inhalation is sometimes preferred over other methods, especially in cases where the goal is weight loss, growth hormone secretion or even balancing emotions.

We are not saying that aromatherapy is like a weight loss cure, but it is a great complimentary therapy to help you prevent overeating and can help you change your relationship with food.

3. Topical application is manifested in baths, massages, compresses and the likes. These in fact form the backbone of the popular perception of Ayurvedic Aromatherapy. Very commonly employed, these means are popularized a great deal by the spa centers and the emerging tourism and hospitality industry. The means employed in topical application are said to ensure and facilitate a healthy blood circulation, pain relief and thereby restoring a stress-free life.

- Hot compresses are no less than a blessing for people susceptible to migraine headaches, sore muscles and sinus headaches. Peppermint oils, rosewood and neroli are recommended in this case. You can follow these remedies from the comforts of your home and see the effect for yourself.

- It follows a simple method to soak a piece of clothing in hot water, which has drops of the essential oil added, and place the cloth on the patient's head, repeating the process. Instant relief is guaranteed.
- A hot bath will not only provide you relaxation but it will also relieve the mucus and replenish your skin. It's not only about relaxation, it can also help you heal skin allergies and improve lymph circulation.

Lemon, cedar wood and rosemary are the perfect, and most commonly used, essential oils employed in massages. They are a great source of getting rid of tension and relieving pain and stress. Massages are the most commonly employed means of spreading the spark of Ayurvedic Aromatherapy. Carrier lotions or oils (called base oils or vegetable oils as mentioned in the previous chapter) assume importance in this case. The most commonly used lotions are almond, Shea and cocoa butter blended with the essential oils to suit the purpose.

You may notice that a lot of the natural and organic lotions and creams that you may be using contain the above aromatic ingredients. These have physical and psychological benefits that can be experienced after a soothing bath. The olfactory senses are triggered and some oils even have the potential to blend in the skin and impart medicinal values by healing the skin of a particular problem.

There are a variety of oils to choose from with different values and a distinct flavor to them. For example, peppermint has exceptional energizing values and lavender is said to be more of a soothing agent. In some cases, lavender is even considered safe without dilution. Do you remember our encounter with mosquitoes in the local woods? We applied a drop of lavender oil on each mosquito bite. Cold packs of essential oils can be used to cure swollen tissues.

Topical application would be more effective if the oils are used in a way to make them stay in longer contact with the skin. The more effectively they are absorbed, more effective they would be in healing. The evaporation of the oils can be prevented by keeping them under a layer of synthetic-free lotion. This enhances penetration. Muscle injuries or injuries in bones and ligaments are more effectively dealt with topical application. The topical method application also works quite well with acupressure.

Back to your base oils, always make sure that they are not minerals oils and are synthetic free. The reason for that is simple; the chemical ingredients create a chemical layer on your skin and prevent the healing essential oils from penetrating it. Such a treatment may of course give you some nice and pleasant aromas for a few seconds or minutes but is really far away from out holistic Ayurvedic aromatherapy.

These three are therefore only different methods to make full use of the bounties of Ayurvedic Aromatherapy. You could easily make a choice and pick the methodology of application best suited to the situation at hand and reap the benefits of Aromatherapy.

Chapter 4: Aromatherapy-Methods

Like other medicinal divisions, Aromatherapy applies its own ingredients and materials that help in the curing process. Some of the common materials employed for practicing and treating with Aromatherapy are as follows:

Essential Oils

We already discussed that essential oils first came into the commercial picture in 1920's, when Rene Maurice Gatttefosse, a French chemist had burned his hand in a laboratory explosion; he used lavender oil. Its antiseptic properties, which delineated from chemical ones, were quite helpful to heal his hand. This drew his attention towards the dermatological aspect of lavender oil and consequently other oils, too. While working in his family's perfume company, he became interested in the antiseptic value of these oils. Eventually, he coined the term *Aromatherepie* and published a book with the same name by 1937.

Later, other French doctors like Jean Valet would use these essential oils in the treatment of soldiers and sometimes to treat psychiatric patients despite much skepticism by other doctors. He continued the work of Gatttefosse in *Aromathérapie*.

Essential oils, compared against their chemical counterparts. are seen to be more responsive and subtle, due to multiple properties that oil constitutes within itself. Chemical ones on the contrary carry within them usually a single property where their sole aim is to fix the problem since they are tailored to do so.

Essential oils have a balancing effect; their sole motive is more than treating a specific problem. It takes the idea of balancing from Ayurveda, which follow the principle of balancing.

These same qualities are followed in case of psychological imbalances such as depression, mood swings, hysteria. For long these have been considered as an excess of one of the humors. Considering this imbalanced state, these essential oils cater to your well being through their fragrance that gives a therapeutic effect to your mind. These are seen as better alternatives than conventional psychotropic drugs. Moreover, human contact while massaging, forms an important extension of Aromatherapy.

It is always advised to use prescribed essential oils and use them in right amounts by consulting an Aroma therapist, since insufficient knowledge can lead to hazardous results. What we offer in this book are simple self-treatments to be performed at home, but if you are on medication or suffer from any serious condition, or are pregnant, we strongly recommend you consult your local Ayurvedic or aromatherapy practitioner first.

Absolutes

As opposed to essential oils, which require steam distillation for preparation, absolutes on the contrary use the method of solvent extraction and enfluerage - a process that uses solid, odorless fats at room temperature in order to capture the fragrance of the plant. These processes are used especially in case of flower petals where there is lesser risk of breaking, unlike distillation.

The process of enfluerage yields a material known as *pomade*, which is a mixture of essential oils and fats, while that of solvent extraction produces a concrete of waxes, fats, essential oils and other plant materials. This pomade and concrete is treated with alcohol in order to extract the absolute.

This absolute which is produced is essentially a highly concentrated, highly-aromatic, oily mixture. This process is usually run at low temperatures so as to avoid breakage of these petals. Since these have high aromatic and therapeutic effects, even a slight concentration of this absolute becomes sufficient. In case of rose absolutes, they solidify when kept at room temperatures, however when they are held in the hand these liquefy.

Often, the usage of absolutes is avoided since it carries with itself a few traces of solvents, even after extraction from the concrete or *pomade*. These can be harmful; however sometimes these are used by Aroma therapists in low quantities.

Carrier Oils

Commonly known as vegetable oils or base oils, carrier oils are used for diluting essential oils and absolute oils for topical application for massages and in Aromatherapy. They absorb the essential oils into the skin. Unlike essential oils, they don't contain any sort of concentrated aroma; however, some oils like olive oil have a mild smell.

These do not evaporate like essential oils, which are volatile. The carrier oils used should be as natural and unadulterated as possible. Cold-pressing and maceration are the two main methods of producing carrier oils. These methods are as follows:

Cold pressed method: In this process you need to make sure that the therapeutic acids and vitamins do not get destroyed. You need to avoid excessive heat for minimizing the changes in the innate properties of the oils.

Maceration: These carrier oils have added properties with respect to its production. In this method, parts of particular plants are cut and mixed with certain carrier oils like olive oil or sunflower oil. This mix is gently stirred for a certain span of time and then stored in a warm area. All the essential oils are then transferred in to the carrier oil and then the macerated mix is carefully filtered, so that the excess plant material can be separated.

You must have noticed that oils used for culinary purposes are often used for massages, which are again economical. Considering the presence of a range of different carrier oils each with various therapeutic properties, the choice of appropriate oil will depend on the area that will be massaged, skin sensitivity and the individual's requirements. Viscosity is a major consideration; for instance, grape seed oil is very thin, while olive oil is much thicker. Sunflower and sweet almond have a viscosity in between.

Infusions

The process of removing the flavors or chemical compounds from the plants in to a solvent like water, alcohol or some sort of oil is called infusion. In this method, it is required to allow the plant material to stay suspended inside the solvent for some time. The resultant liquid is called as the infusion.

The plant materials are used as dry herbs, berries or flowers. The liquid (oil, water or alcohol) is boiled to the right temperature and then dispensed on the herb. The liquid is either strained to remove the plants, or the herbs are separated from the liquid. The infusion is then refrigerated or bottled for later use.

Phytoncides

Phytoncides are antimicrobial chemical compounds that are derived from plants. Coined by Russian Biochemist, Dr. Boris P Tokin, Phytoncides literally mean, "something that is exterminated from the plant". As per Dr. Tokin, certain plants excrete active ingredients that prevent them from being eaten by insects and from rotting.

Some good examples of Phytoncides are spice, garlic, onion, oak tree, tea tree and pine tree. These substances defend the plants from bacterial and fungal growth.

Chapter 5: Popular Oils

Aromatherapy employs a lot of different fragrant oils that have healing and soothing properties. You will notice that most of them are made from commonly used herbs and flowers. Let's dive into it!

Thyme Oil

Thyme oil is reddish-brown to amber in color and has a sweet and strong herbal smell. It is extracted from steam or distillation of the fresh/partly dried flowering tops and leaves of the thyme plant. It was used in ancient times by the Greeks, the Romans, and the Egyptians for medicinal purposes.

The oil derives its name from the Greek word 'thymos' which means 'perfume' which is related to its use as incense in Greek temples. The Egyptians also used it in the embalming process.

Thyme oil is found to strengthen the nerves and enhance concentration and memory. It is also recommended as a natural remedy for the following conditions:

- Depression
- Colds
- Catarrh
- Sinusitis
- Sore throat
- Tonsillitis

Thyme has a warming effect on the area of application and is also helpful in treating:

- Poor circulation
- Muscular aches

- Sprains
- Obesity and edema
- Irregular periods
- Cellulite

It is a natural antiseptic; we always use it in winter to prevent colds and flu.

Thyme oil blends particularly well with lemon, grapefruit, bergamot, rosemary, pine and lavender.

Peppermint Oil

A native to the Mediterranean, the pale yellow peppermint oil has a fresh and sharp, menthol-like smell. It is extracted from a perennial herb that has slight, saw-like leaves and pink/mauve flowers. It is extracted using the steam distillation method from the body of the plant (either fresh or partly dried) that is on the surface of the ground before flowering.

This herb has many species and this might produce varieties of the oil with slight differences. Peppermint piperita is a hybrid of two such sub-species, spearmint (M. spicata) and watermint (M. aquatica).

Peppermint oil is excellent for several skin related problems like skin irritation, itchiness, skin redness due to inflammation (in which case the cooling effect of the oil on skin helps). It is used for acne, dermatitis, scabies, ringworm and pruritus, and also for relieving itching or sunburn.

Peppermint oil provides the natural cure for a range of problems related to the digestive system for example:

- Cramps
- Nausea
- Colic

- flatuence

It also helps in relieving pain in cases of:

- toothache,
- neuralgia,
- rheumatism,
- menstrual cramps,
- foot ache and other muscular pains.

The effect of peppermint oil on the mind is observed in its ability to refresh the spirit and stimulate mental agility. It relieves the mind of fatigue and depression and also improves concentration.

I, James, always have some peppermint essential oil in my office. When I feel like I get stuck with a project, I use it with my diffuser, or sometimes I take a 15 minute break for a mini self-massage. I mix 2 drops of peppermint oil with a teaspoon of coconut oil and I massage my neck and my ears. It helps me refresh and very often calm down my vita-pita tendencies.

Benzoin, lemon, rosemary, lavender, marjoram and eucalyptus are some of the oils that blend well with peppermint oil.

Elena really enjoys blending peppermint oil with cinnamon oil- we both think it's a greatly stimulating aphrodisiac and we recommend you try it with your partner.

Peppermint also makes an amazing blend with citric scents, like for example bergamot, verbena, lemon, or sweet orange. We find such blends suitable for both if us, even though we are different doshas. While a peppermint scent is cooling and refreshing (perfect for people with pitta tendencies who get angry and red easily!), citrus scents are slightly uplifting (great for kaphas who have tendency to get stuck or even lazy). Of course, we are making it really general now, but we hope you get the way it works. We also encourage you to try aromatherapy and work on balancing your dosha, and most importantly, understanding practicing and feeling it

Lavandula Oil

An extract of Lavandula Augustifolia, Lavandula oil is more popularly known as lavender oil. This oil has a clear color along with watery viscosity. It has a fresh aroma and has been used in bath routines since the ancient times among the Romans.

Lavandula oil has a very soothing effect. It revitalizes and tones different types of skin issues like oily skin, acne, burns, boils, insect bites, lice, and stings.

You can use it as mosquito repellant. It also has the capacity to relax the nerves, to relieve tension, panic, depression, hysteria, migraines, headaches and insomnia.

It helps with several ailments related to the digestive system (vomiting, nausea, colic and flatulence) and the respiratory system (asthma, colds, throat infections, halitosis, whooping coughs, laryngitis and bronchitis).

Lavandula oil is also beneficial in relieving pain in cases of arthritis, rheumatism, lumbago and muscular pains, especially those related to sporting activities.

Lavender oil particularly blends well with other oils like pine, geranium, all kinds of citrus oils, clary sage and cedar wood.

Jasmine Oil

Jasmine essential oil has a sweet and floral smell. It is extracted from the white-star shaped flowers of the jasmine shrubs which are evergreen, fragile creepers that can grow up to 10 meters. It is picked at night when its aroma is at its peak. Jasmine oil has been used for medicinal purposes since the ancient times by the Chinese, Indians and the Arabians. It was also used as an aphrodisiac as well as for other ceremonial purposes.

Because of its soothing floral smell, it produces a feeling of euphoria, confidence and optimism. It soothes the nerves, overcomes the feelings of depression and revitalizes and restores energy. Again because of its deeply calming nature, jasmine oil helps with a number of sexual problems such as premature ejaculation, impotency and frigidity (hence, its ancient use is as of aphrodisiac).

This oil is non-toxic, non-irritant and generally also non-sensitizing. Thus, it does not show any side-effects. However, some people might have an allergic reaction to jasmine oil. The therapeutic properties of jasmine oil which determines its various applications are aphrodisiac, antiseptic, anti-depressant, anti-spasmodic, expectorant, cicatrisant, parturient, galactagogue, uterine and sedative.

Jasmine oil is a great natural remedy for sensitive and greasy complexions. Aside from facial treatments, ayurvedic spas use it to reduce stretch marks.

Jasmine oil has a very beneficial effect on ailments related to the respiratory system. It soothes irritating coughs and helps with laryngitis and hoarseness.

The essential oils that Jasmine oil blends particularly well with are rose, bergamot, sandalwood and all citrus oils.

Chapter 6: Using Ayurvedic Aromatherapy for Common Ailments

Oils used in Aromatherapy can be absorbed through the pores in your skin or through the nose. Oils are easily sensed by the receptors in your nose, which carry it to the brain with the help of neurons. Often the oils are applied to the palms of the hand or the bottom of the feet from where they are absorbed into the blood stream in less than five minutes.

Acne

There is an array of essential oils that can help you control and prevent the problem of acne. Aromatherapy not just clears the skin but does it by helping the management of the very underlying problems that cause acne. They regulate the oil production by the oil glands under the skin, balance hormones and regulate fluctuations, reduce stress, and improve the complexion.

This is why Aromatherapy is the ideal treatment for your acne problems like pimples, blemishes, and other types of skin eruptions. This is the reason why even chemical products in the market claim to have been inspired by an Ayurvedic formula containing essential oils such as eucalyptus oil, lemon or lavender. Essential oils are also effective in fighting off bacteria from the acne affected region.

The best essential oils for acne treatment are:

- eucalyptus
- geranium

- wood
- sandalwood
- lemongrass
- frankincense
- lavender
- tree
- clary sage
- juniper berry
- lemon
- bergamot
- verbena

Base oils recommended for anti-acne treatments are hazelnut oil, coconut oil as well as aloe vera gel (this one has a really nice, light consistency and is perfect for hot summers).

Addiction

Lately, Aromatherapy has become a popular therapeutic practice in treating the withdrawal symptoms during a drug addiction treatment. Though varying according to the addiction of drug, withdrawal symptoms generally include sleep disturbances, restlessness, irritability and anxiety. Essential oils used in Aromatherapy help to create an emotional balance, promoting a sense of calm by reducing the feelings of stress. The result of this is a considerable reduction in several withdrawal symptoms.

Aromatherapy is mostly used as an adjunct to support the traditional addiction treatment methods. Aromatherapy, when combined with massage therapy, considerably improves the therapeutic value of the latter. It produces a greater sense of holistic well-being because of an increased sense of relaxation and healing of pain.

Below listed are some of the Aromatherapy essential oils that are especially beneficial in treatment of withdrawal symptoms:

1. **Anise Aromatherapy:** Anise curbs cravings for chocolate or sugary items, which are often experienced by those fighting alcohol addictions. It also relieves stress and induces better sleep and provides relaxation.

2. **Chamomile Aromatherapy:** Chamomile has been traditionally regarded as an antidepressant. It helps to relieve suppressed anger, and thus provides relaxation and aids sleep. Helpful in fighting cravings and addictions

3. **Frankincense Aromatherapy:** Frankincense induces spirituality, clears perception, and leads to higher states of consciousness. It encourages a kind of optimism and also helps in a release from the past. It is also effective in combating cravings for sugar or sedatives.

4. **Lavender Aromatherapy:** Lavender provides relief from lethargy and exhaustion due to work, calms the nerves, thus helping during the withdrawal phase. It also reduces cravings for alcohol.

5. **Fennel Aromatherapy:** Fennel also helps in dispelling cravings for chocolate, alcohol and sugar, common during the withdrawal phase.

Alzheimer's disease and other forms of dementia

Yes, it may sound quite surprising but it is true, Aromatherapy plays an important role in treating dementia and Alzheimer's disease to a great extent. People suffering from Alzheimer's disease or other forms of dementia frequently experience states of agitation that makes them a challenge to their family or caregivers.

Traditional medication involves the use of strong tranquilizers that suppress such feelings of agitation, but it is generally accompanied by partial or full unconsciousness of the patient. Thus, Ayurvedic Aromatherapy becomes an important form of alternative medication in which essential oils are applied to the patients through methods like massage, direct inhalation, bath, ambient diffusion etc.

Different essential oils show varying properties. Some popular and easily available essential oils used in the medication of dementia include:

Lavender: It is an antidepressant which calms the nerves and balances strong emotions. It is also good for insomnia, thus, promoting better sleep and a better overall mood.

Rosemary: Rosemary essential oil stimulates body and mind, creating a feeling of emotional well-being. It also improves the cognitive performance of the mind in its accuracy and also in terms of speed.

Peppermint: When used in the morning, it boosts appetite. It stimulates the mind and calms the nerves. It is also helpful in keeping a check on absent-mindedness caused by dementia.

Lemon Balm: It induces a feeling of calmness and relaxation and is very effective in cases of anxiety and insomnia.

Chapter 7: Ayurvedic Spa at Home

In order to select an essential oil, an Aroma therapist carefully studies the patient, which includes his lifestyle, eating pattern, emotional and behavioral pattern. This is known as a holistic examination in Aromatherapy. Keeping this approach in mind, in correspondence to *doshas*, various essential oils are recommended.

We encourage you to be your own patient.

We have included a bonus chapter. We recommend you have a look at our mini dosha test.

We think that discovering your prevalent dosha is really exciting; it's like getting to know yourself. You can also do the test with your family and friends.

These are just the general examples as for some oils that your dosha may like:

- *Vata* **likes** ginger, cinnamon, camphor, rosewood, anise, angelica, lemon, eucalyptus and basil
- *Pitta* *likes* chamomile, yarrow, lime, coriander, sandalwood, and peppermint.
- *Kapha likes* sage, rosemary, naiouli, and clove

Considering the three basic body types, it is necessary to know the 'imbalance' caused due to excess of any of the *doshas*.

For example, if you experience anger, ulcers and agitation, you should try to balance pitta, and therefore should choose oils that pita dosha likes (calming and relaxing).

Vata

- Symptoms: In this, you are susceptible to headaches, nervous anxiety, hypersensitivity, dry skin, and constipation.
- Precautions: Avoid sharp-perfumed essential oils.
- Sources: Warm and stimulating oils like camphor, cypress and cinnamon, along with calming and stabilizing oils like jasmine, rose, sandalwood are blended in sesame oil, as it has the ability to penetrate in to the skin.

Pitta

- Symptoms: Ulcers, acidity, fevers, agitation, inflammatory skin diseases and anger
- Sources: Oils that give a cooling effect usually with fragrances of flowers like jasmine, gardenia, rose, mint and sandalwood, which are blended in to a cooling carrier oil like coconut oil.

Kapha

- Symptoms: Respiratory ailments
- Sources: Oils that have a warm effect like basil, cedar, pine and sage. Sharp fragrances that have a stimulating effect can also be beneficial.

AYURVEDIC SPA TIPS FOR VATA:

Self-Massage (self- Abhy, or: Abhyanga) for vattas that need more focus, balance and warmth to balance their dosha.

You can get back on track, relax, rejuvenate and detoxify with the following oils that we recommend:

VEGETABLE BASE OILS:

- Coconut oil
- Jojoba oil
- Almond oil
- Safflower oil
- Sesame Oil

ESSENTIAL OILS:

- Basil (James loves it, we have mentioned it before, haven't we?)
- Patchouli
- Vetiver

The proportion for a full body massage is more or less:

2 tablespoons of your chosen vegetable oil + about 10 drops (in total) of your chosen essential oil (or oils if you blend more than 1).

If you are new to aromatherapy or to particular oils, we suggest you test your blend on a small area of skin, for example on your forearm.

Now, since James is quite tall and athletic and he does not shave his legs or chest, he needs more oils (about 3 tablespoons + 15 drops of essential oils).

Elena, on the other hand is small and thin. She does shave her legs, haha and does not have any hair on her chest yet this is why she can do with small amount of oils, like for example: 1 tablespoon + 5 drops of her chosen essential oils (she loves 2 drops of bergamot + 3 drops of mint, great for her kapha nature.

Additionally, we recommend you use stones for self-massage. It's very easy, just press the points on your body where the tension is. For example, James tends to accumulate tension in his neck. This happens after long hours of writing as well as emotional stress that he may sometimes fall victim of. If you are vatta, simply touch and press the affected areas with one or more of the following stones:

- Tiger eye
- Lapis Lazuli (also for pitas, great for insomnia and restlessness, if you are a workaholic, you have just found your stone)
- Emerald
- Cat's eye
- Amethyst

You can also sleep with them. Yes! Put them under the pillow or on your night table. You can also meditate with them, carry them in your bad or keep them in your office. Wash them regularly with cold water and sea salt so as to purify their energy field. They will heal and balance your chakras and result in your ultimate wellness!

Vatta people, like for example James, are very creative. They put their heart and soul into their work. This is why they very often feel burnt out and as a result experience lack of energy and even anxiousness and nervousness.

This is why we recommend you get some highly therapeutic ayurvedic herbs and infusions and use them in your health spa. Don't drink coffee nor back tea. It will only aggravate your condition. There is a range of vata friendly and balancing drinks:

- cinnamon bark,
- chicory root, organic
- ginger root,
- cardamom,
- nutmeg

- mint
- chamomile

You can use them separately or mix them.

James likes to relax in a nice, warm bath with aromatherapy (he likes basil, as you already know, but he also likes sweet calming and grounding scents like: rose, angelica, bergamot (Elena loves it too), chamomile and vanilla.

We also both think that ylang ylang is a great idea for a nice and warm bath for two! It is an aphrodisiac, so be careful!

Simply add a few drops of your chosen essential oil or oils to your bath when the water is not running. Remember to stir the water energetically before you jump in- you want to make sure that essential oils are equally distributed.

So, while relaxing in his bath, James likes to enjoy his ayrvedic herbs and herbal teas. Before discovering Ayurveda, James used to resort to alcohol and drugs (bad idea!) and these would only aggravate his vata condition (he has pitta tendencies also which means that he can hit the roof easily).

Does he want to go back to where he was before?

No, because ayurvedic sensation of "feeling good" is just awesome!

AYURVEDIC SPA TIPS FOR KAPHA:

If you are kapha, you may need some holistic treatments to get your inspiration back and put you back on track. No slacking off!

Now you know the procedure of self-massage. If you are kapha, like Elena (if you are still unsure, check out the BONUS chapter, and follow our dosha test, it's fun!) your body and mind will be grateful for a regular self-massage with one or more of the following oils (you already know that essential oils must be first diluted in a vegetable base oil, so let's get straight to the point!).

Vegetable Oils:

- coconut oil
- mustard seed (really energizing) oil
- almond oil
- grape seed oil

(Elena recommends it for facial treatments, it is a natural anti-wrinkle treatment)

Essential Oils:

- Bergamot
- Lemon
- Pepper Mint
- Juniper
- Fennel
- Allspice
- Cinnamon
- Clove
- Lime
- Marjoram
- Thyme
- Myrrh
- Myrtle

Additional Therapies

Stones for self-massage, meditation and balancing for kapha people:

- Coral
- Sunstone
- Red Jasper
- Garnet

Herbs that we recommend if you tend to have kapha properties (lack of motivation, laziness, lack of productive energy, overeating, weight gain, oversleeping, and toxin accumulation-what a marvelous combination! Luckily, we know how to get to the root of the problem with ayurvedic aromatherapy and ayurvedic herbal infusions):

- Allspice
- Black pepper
- Rosemary
- Cinammon
- Coriander
- Turmeric

In short, we want something spicy, sexy and invigorating. This is what kaphas need.

Now, you may be tempted to drink coffe. You are probably thinking: "hey, if I am Kapha I need to wake up. Where is my mega cup of morning coffee?".

This is what we used to think as well, and if you ask Elena, she used to be a coffee addict...Unfortunately, what goes up must go down (even faster). Around midday Elena would suffer from horrible headaches and migraines. She would feel even more tired. This is why she finally learned how to listen to her amazing body and give it what it needs- natural, herbal stimulation that was designed for her dosha by the Mother Nature!

Kapha people tend to suffer from slow metabolism and usually have it difficult to lose weight. Include the mix of herbal infusions that we suggested and you will be amazed at the results.

If you suffer from toxin accumulation, fat accumulation and water retention, then do your daily Abhyanga and create your internal pharmacy with the following essential oils:

- Grapefruit
- Peppermint
- Juniper
- Fennel

You should focus on your stomach area.

The blend that Elena loves is the following:

- 1 tablespoon of coconutoil
- 4 drops of rosemary essential oil
- 2 drops of pepper mint essential oil
- 2 drops of lemon essential oil
- 2 drops of grapefruit essential oil
- 1 drop of frankincense essential oil

Apply on your belly and legs. Use energetic frictions and rub the area. You want to go as red as you can to stimulate your internal detoxifying energy that has been dormant for years!

If you suffer from constipation, massage your stomach and lumbar area with the following mix (perform 3 times a day, 2 hours after your meal):

- 1 tablespoon of your chosen vegetable oil
- 2 drops of peppermint oil
- 2 drops of clove
- 2 drops of allspice

- 2 drops of sweet orange oil

AYURVEDIC SPA TIPS FOR PITTA

The biggest obstacle that pitta people are facing is to keep calm, don't get that revved up, and to be patient. Things can sort themselves out naturally, there is no need to be such a control freak and have everyone do what you say.

We hope that you get this comparison! Pitta people have also tendency to work too much. While ayurveda is not the ultimate workaholism cure and much more work is needed on the mental level, ayurvedic aromatherapy and other natural therapies can soothe pitas and give them some well-deserved rest.

Like we said, pitas are always on fire. When under stress, they tend to work even harder. One of our best friends, John, is the most "pitta-like" person we have ever met. Everything in him is pitta, both his looks and his character. Not long ago, he was going through a painful divorce and he felt depressed. Now, here is a big difference between people that are kapha and people that are pitta. Kapha people, when depressed, tend to stay in and lead a life as a recluse. Pittas, on the other hand, get suckered into a whirl of work and intense partying and socializing. Both of these patterns are unbalancing and destroying.

Luckily, John is now recovered and back on track. In fact, he started dating again. His new girlfriend is also pitta and they are now both learning how to balance their explosive natures. They want their relationship to last, and two pitas on fire are a great match for a Latin telenovela, but not for a peaceful and balanced relationship that both John and his new partner seek...

People like John need calming, soothing and rejuvenating ayurvedic spa daily.

The tips that our friend is following now, include, of course the following ayurvedic natural therapies:

Self-Massage (do you remember how it is called in Ayurveda…? If you don't, then you have something of an absent-minded vata quality in you…!)

Vegetable Oils:

- Coconut oil (this one is the most famous one, come on, everyone loves coconut oil, it's like a living legend!)
- Sunflower
- Olive
- Almond

Essential Oils:

- Lavender
- Lavandin
- Chamomile
- Geranium
- Lemongrass
- Yatamansi
- Sandalwood (this one is really popular at ayurvedic health spas)

Stones:

- Lapis
- Yade
- Perdiot
- Pearl
- Emerald

Anger is an energy vampire. The more you hit the roof, the more tired you will feel. We suggest you try to cool down and chill out with the following herbal infusions:

- Spearmint
- Corriander

They seem to be working perfectly for John!

Now, it wasn't easy to convince John to get started on ayurveda. You see, typical pitas are really stubborn and set in their ways. They also tend to overindulge in foods that are not necessarily good for them (can be also alcohol, drugs and smoking- bad combination!). This is why they easily inflammable nature and very often bad habits result in digestive problems (acidity, ulcers). If this is something you are prone to, take action with your ayurvedic spa. Drink your soothing infusions daily and treat yourself to an aromatic massage. You can also ask your partner. John and his new girlfriend got really hooked on aromatherapy now! It's also a great time to develop intimacy with your partner. So much better than just watching TV (We don't recommend it, unless you want to kill your sex life forever!).

Here are some super soothing and relaxing blends for full-body massage for pitas.

Chill out Pitta Blend dedicated to our inspiring friend, John:

- 2 tablespoons of coconut oil
- 3 drops of Sandalwoodessential oil
- 5 drops of Lavender essential oil
- 3 drops of Chamomile essential oil

Apply as a full body massage.

If you feel like on the verge of hitting the roof, massage your face, forehead and scalp with the following blend:

- 1 tablespoon of your chosen vegetable oil
- 2 drops of peppermint essential oil
- 2 drops of geranium essential oil
- 2 drops of coriander essential oil

Massage gently for about 15 minutes. Breathe in and out. Leave in for about an hour. This is also a fantastic treatment to make your hair follicles stronger and so your hair- healthier.

This brings us to another healthy ayurvedic spa ritual.

Let's get started on our HOLISTIC HAIR SPA inspired by Ayurvedic Head Massage!

We both think that nowadays people use too many chemical shampoos and too many conditioners. It's both expensive and unhealthy. Back in India we did training in Indian Head Massage and we fell in love with this therapy. We will surely write a book on ayurvedic self-massage techniques, but for now we will only focus on aromatherapy that you can use both to improve your hair condition and to achieve deep, **holistic state of relaxation**.

We do this treatment at least twice a week.

The rules are very simple: before you wash your hair, apply your chosen oils on your scalp and massage energetically. Try to move the scalp as much as possible; the oils are full of nutrients that are excellent for hair follicles. They also penetrate and nourish the hair and can even treat the split ends.

You can either do this treatment 1 hour before washing your hair (it's good to massage your head for at least 15 minutes and then keep the oils for at least half an hour) or you can do it at nighttime and wash your hair the following day. We really recommend this treatment for damaged hair.

How to blend the oils?

We recommend that you use about 2 tablespoons of your chosen vegetable oil and up to 20 drops of your chosen essential oil, or oils if you are blending more than 1.

Vegetable oils for head massage

Choose your vegetable oil according to your dosha. We really love: coconut oil, sesame Oil and sweet almond oil.

Then, personalize your blend using essential oils depending on your hair type and possible conditions you want to eliminate.

You can also add a few drops of your chosen essential oil to your organic shampoo or, if you are using one, to your organic conditioner. The effect will be spectacular- super strong, healthy and shiny hair!

OILY HAIR-chamomile, grapefruit, lemongrass, lemon

DRY HAIR-ylang ylang, rosewood, sandalwood, palmarosa

STIMULATE HAIR GROWTH-rosemary, juniper, grapefruit

FIGHT DANDRUFF AND ITCHY SCALP-bergamot, tea tree, orange

DAMAGED, BLEACHED OR COLORED HAIR THAT NEEDS HEALING-sandalwood, ylang ylang, patchouli,

NORMAL HAIR THAT WANTS TO BE TREATED NATURALLY-geranium, lavender, ylang ylang

Additionaly we recommend you use herbal teas and supplements that contain aloe vera and clivers herb- these are excellent to prevent hair loss and stimulate hair growth.

Of course, it's not only about head and scalp massage. We suggest you use your massage time as time for reflection and meditation. Breathe in and out deeply. Massage your neck and your shoulders. Stretch intuitively and breathe in the wonderful and healing aromas.

You can also do it with your partner. It's really relaxing and therapeutic.

Below you will find a few recipes that we love using on a regular basis.

Decongesting steam

While in the winter, some coughing and sniffles can be an irritant. Tea tree oil has powerful antiviral, combined with the potency of eucalyptus oil, which will help in decongesting the lungs and sinuses.

Ingredients
-4 cups boiling water

-5 drops eucalyptus essential oil (peppermint can also be used)

-5 drops tea tree essential oil

Process:
Boil the water in a teakettle. As soon as it comes to a boil, pour it into a large-enough container. Once this is done, mix the essential oils into it, and cover with a towel. Lift the towel and place your face so that your nose and mouth are only a few inches from the concoction. Take a couple of long and deep breaths, but make sure you spread a towel over your head.

Homemade Teething oil

Clove is a natural analgesic used in dentistry.

Ingredients
-2 tablespoons of olive oil, for a mild flavor 1 tablespoon of olive oil and 1 tablespoon of coconut oil.

-2-3 drops of clove bud essential oil

Process:
Combine the ingredients and taste it to make sure that it's not too strong. Then pour the mixture in a clean container. Since light oxidizes oil, use a dark amber container.

Use:
Make sure that the clove is absolutely diluted before application. Shake the mixture well and apply it on the gums with the fingertips. Reapply every 1-2 hours, as required.

Warming Chest Rub

Ingredients
-4 tsp Almond Oil

-4 tbsp Beeswax Pellets

-1 tbsp Coconut Butter

-30 drops Eucalyptus Oil

-10 drops Thyme Oil

-10 drops Tea Tree Oil

Process:
-In a glass bowl over boiling water, heat the almond oil, beeswax pellets, and coconut butter until melted. Remove the bowl from heat and let it sit for 60 seconds, keep stirring it to avoid solidification. Mix in essential oils, and pour them into a jar. Wait until the mixture has completely cooled before putting the cap on.

-When ready for use, rub a quarter sized portion between your fingers before placing on the child's (or your) chest or under the nose.

-Store this in a cool dark area for up to 1 month.

BONUS CHAPTER

DOSHA TEST

Hey, congratulations for going through his book to the very end.

Now, here comes the fan part- discovering yourself and learning more about your tendencies, strengths and weakness. This is really holistic stuff!

After doing this test you will know you prevalent dosha. Sometimes it might be even two doshas. Then, we suggest you start to observe your body, mind and emotions. If you want to take it to a new level, start your ayurvedic holistic diary.

Here's what you should include:

-How you feel today- your body, mind, feelings, emotions

-What body work have you done today

-What have you eaten

-Spices and herbs you have used

-Your spa treatments

This is how you will be able to notice certain patterns and emotions and how they influence your wellness. Once you discover that, you will be in the minority of Westerners who practice mindful and holistic self-care.

This process can also be abundant in errors. Don't worry about it. As long as you observe, learn and gradually eliminate negative habits from your lifestyle, you will be elbowing your way towards your health and wellbeing. Just like you have ever wanted!

For now just relax and do the test. Have a look which qualities prevail. This will be your prevalent dosha. Remember that no one is ever 100% vata, pitta or kapha. The tendencies and features mix and overlap. We also change and do our own holistic evolution.

Still, certain qualities are pre-born. For example some people are prone to colds, some people are prone to hair loss and some people are prone to weight gain. However, this does not mean that they should just sit with their arms crossed and not doing anything. Once should fight to at least try to improve their overall health. This is what oriental medicine is all about.

VATA

BODY TYPE- slim, light, fragile

HEIGHT-very tall or very short

WEIGHT-slim, light body weight. Veins and bones easily visible and marked.

SKIN-dry, sensitive, cold, sunburns easily

HAIR-dry, dandruff, very often brown or black

FACE-early wrinkles, small features,

EYES- small, dry, instable, dark

LIPS-slim, small, dry, can tremble easily

TEETH-small, there are spaces between them

CHEST-small, slim

HANDS- cold, dry, shaky. You can see veins and the bones mark easily.

NAILS-small, dry, cracked

FEET-large, dry, narrow

VOICE-speaks a lot, silent, soft, speaks fast

SLEEP-light, easily awaken, insomniac tendency

URINE-no color, does not urinate often

FECES- dry, easily constipated

PERSPIRATION-changeable, no strong odor, does not perspire a lot

APETITE-does not eat a lot, appetite changes depending on mood, when stressed does not eat

THIRST- changeable

CIRCULATION- poor, sluggish

ACTIVITY AND ENERGY-hyperactive, fast, likes to keep busy, very active

SENSITIVITY-hates cold, heat and wind

STAMINA AND STRENGTH-little stamina but can change, normally gets easily tired after excessive stamina workouts

DISEASES- TENDENCIES-arthritis, insomnia, nervousness, anxiety, mental imbalances

NEUROTIC TEMDEMCIES-anxiety, shakiness

POSITIVE MENTAL FEATURES-creative, active, enthusiastic, with imagination, motivating and motivated, encouraging, flexible

NEGATIVE MENTAL FEATURES-often in two minds, oversensitive, concerned about what other say.

SCORED....OUT OF 27

PITTA:

BODY TYPE- medium, quite strong

HEIGHT- medium

WEIGHT- medium, moderated, muscular

SKIN-red, humid, oily, beauty spots and freckles, can sun burn easily, can be prone to acne

HAIR-usually blonde or ginger, light colors. Quite thin and fragile. Prone to baldness and premature white hair.

FACE- reddish, tendency to get wrinkles on the forehead <but not always), very sharp features

EYES-light colors, sensitive, go read easily, penetrating, don't tolerate excess sun

LIPS-medium, red, soft

TEETH- medium, difficult to maintain them white (yellow tendencies), gums have tendency to bleed easily

CHEST-medium size

HANDS- warm, wet, medium, red

NAILS- have pinkish color, medium, soft

FEET-medium, soft, pinkish

VOICE-likes discussions and arguments, high-pitched, penetrating, strong

SLEEP- sleeps quite well but can wake up at night, usually able to get back to sleep again

URINE-abundant, yellow, red, warm

FECES- diarrhea tendency, goes to a bathroom a lot!

PERSPIRATION-abundant, strong odor, warm

APETITE- good digestion and excellent appetite, tends to overindulge in eating, drinking etc,

THIRST-strong, excessive, craves water all the time

CIRCULATION- strong, warm

ACTIVITY AND ENERGY- motivated, goal-orientated, with a plan to follow, well-organized, workaholic

SENSITIVITY-Fire, sun, heat- can't stand them, gets irritated

STAMINA AND STRENGTH-good stamina

DISEASES- TENDENCIES-fever, inflammation, infection

NEUROTIC TEMDEMCIES-anger, jealousy

POSITIVE MENTAL FEATURES-intelligent, competitive, very focused and centered

NEGATIVE MENTAL FEATURES- aggressive, irritable, easily frustrated

SCORED....OUT OF 27

KAPHA:

BODY TYPE- big, chubby, thick

HEIGHT-tall and husky or small and chubby

WEIGHT-excess weight

SKIN-arm, soft, oily, pale complexion

HAIR-wavy, curly, strong, fizzy, dark or light

FACE-big features, rounded

EYES-white, calm, attractive

LIPS-big, humid, firm

TEETH- white, big, strong

CHEST- big, strong

HANDS-big, oily, cold

NAILS-big, soft, white, strong

FEET-big, wide

VOICE-nice,- slow, does not talk a lot

SLEEP- hard to wake up!

URINE-white in color, moderate amounts

FECES-slow or moderate, solid

PERSPIRATION-moderate, cold

APETITE-uses food to escape from problems, if balanced, eats well, moderate amounts

THIRST does not drink too much

CIRCULATION- slow and steady

ACTIVITY AND ENERGY- slow, lazy, lethargic, can't motivate for action

SENSITIVITY-hates cold and humidity

STAMINA AND STRENGTH-good stamina, fit

DISEASES- TENDENCIES-water retention, overweight, respiratory system, runny nose

NEUROTIC TEMDEMCIES-does not feel like taking action, lethargic

POSITIVE MENTAL FEATURES-calm, steady, realistic

NEGATIVE MENTAL FEATURES- reluctant to change, stubborn, very sentimental

SCORED....OUT OF 27

Now do the math again...what's your prevalent dosha?

Conclusion

We have tried to provide you with the most pragmatic usage of Ayurvedic Aromatherapy so as to allow you to use their multiple combined benefits for a healthier and more energetic life. By using the methods described in this booklet, you can get started on aromatherapy in a holistic, Ayurvedic and personalized way.

Of course, this is only the beginning of your journey. We encourage you to study, explore and investigate and commit yourself to becoming a student of Ayurveda and gain a better and more balanced quality of life.

We hope that you are now on your way to discovering the multiple facets of Ayurvedic Aromatherapy and that you will be enjoying the immediate relief that it can provide you with!

You may also be interested in checking out our other book and learning more about Ayurveda and holistic healing:

Free Complimentary PDF eBook +

Wellness Newsletter

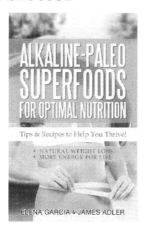

Download link:

www.holisticwellnessbooks.com/bonus

Problems with your download?

Contact us: elenajamesbooks@gmail.com

Welcome to Holistic Wellness Books family!

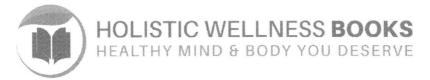

Follow us on Facebook & Twitter and be the first one to get free and bargain eBook and other holistic resources!

Click on the images below or visit:

www.twitter.com/Wellness_Books

www.facebook.com/HolisticWellnessBooks

Wishing you all the best on your Ayurvedic Aromatherapy journey!

Elena and James

www.amazon.com/author/elenagarcia

Made in the USA
Columbia, SC
15 December 2019